To Comfort Always: A Nurse's Guide to End of Life Care

Linda Norlander, RN, MS

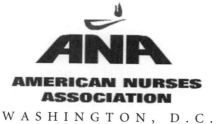

AMERICAN NURSES ASSOCIATION

WASHINGTON, D.C.

Library of Congress Cataloging-in-Publication Data

Norlander, Linda, 1949-
To comfort always: a nurse's guide to end of life care/ Linda Norlander.
    p. ; cm.
    Includes bibliographical references and index.
    ISBN 1-55810-177-2
1. Terminal care. 2. Terminally ill–Care. 3. Nursing. 4. Palliative treatment. I. Title.
[DNLM: 1. Terminal Care–methods. 2. Nursing Care–methods.
WY 152 N841w2001]
RT87.T45. N674 2001
616.029-dc21

2001053545

Cover photograph ("Lone Elm") by Jerry Mathiason is reproduced
by permission of the photographer.

Published by
American Nurses Publishing
600 Maryland Avenue, SW
Suite 100 West
Washington, DC 20024-2571
ISBN 1-55810-177-2
EOL21   1.5 M   11/01

Acknowledgements

I want to express my thanks and gratitude to the people who assisted me in putting this book together. First and foremost, to Kerstin McSteen, RN, MS, CHPN—a great hospice and palliative care nurse and a wonderful friend. To Jody Chrastek, RN, MS, for her guidance on care for children. To Jane O'Brien, MA, for her guidance on chapter organization and on cultural sensitivity. To Barry Baines, MD, co-chair of the Minnesota Commission on End of Life Care, for his work on the Five Guiding Principles. To Claude Webb, RN, for his hospice expertise. To Rosanne O'Connor and Eric Wurzbacher from ANA Publishing, for believing in this project. And finally, to my husband Jerome Norlander, for his support over all the weekends when I was "missing in action" to write this book.

Contents

Foreword: I Didn't Know What I Didn't Know   *ix*

Chapter 1: Where to Begin   *1*
    Guiding Principles of End of Life Care   *1*
    Core Nursing Responsibilities: Skilled Clinician, Advocate, and Guide   *2*
    What Do Patients and Families Want for Care at the End of Life?   *3*
    When Do We Start Providing End of Life Care?   *4*
    A Team Approach   *5*
    Summary   *6*
    References and Other Resources   *7*

Chapter 2: Choices At the End of Life: Advance Care Planning   *9*
    The Courageous Conversation   *9*
    Skilled Clinician: Understanding the Elements of Advance Care Planning   *10*
    Advance Directives   *12*
    Advocating in Advance Care Planning: Making Sure Wishes are Honored   *13*
    Guiding in Advance Care Planning: Recognizing the Common Barriers   *13*
    Common Questions Patients Ask About Advance Directives   *15*
    Summary   *16*
    References and Other Resources   *16*

Chapter 3: Pain Management: It's More Than Knowing the Meds   *19*
    Listening to the Patient's Pain   *19*
    Skilled Clinician: Assessment and Managment of Pain   *20*
    Use of Adjuvant Medications   *23*
    Advocating: Assuring That the Patient's Pain Relief Goals are Met   *24*
    Guiding Patients and Families: Addressing Common Myths   *25*
    Know the Resources   *26*

Summary   *27*
References and Other Resources   *27*

Chapter 4: Physical Symptom Management: Knowing What to Look For   29
Common Symptoms   *29*
Skilled Clinician: Assessment and Management of Common Symptoms   *30*
Advocating: Linking the Needs of the Patient and Family
    to the Medical System   *35*
Guiding Patients and Families: Preparing, Listening, and Assuring   *36*
Summary   *36*
References and Other Resources   *37*

Chapter 5: Suffering: It's Not Just the Pain   39
What is Suffering at the End of Life?   *39*
Skilled Clinician: Assessing Suffering   *40*
Advocating for Patients: Assuring a Holistic View   *42*
Guiding Patients and Families: Start with Yourself   *43*
Summary   *45*
References and Other Resources   *45*

Chapter 6: Active Dying: The Final Days and Hours   47
Active Dying: What Does It Mean?   *47*
Skilled Clinician: Assessing and Intervening When Death is Near   *47*
Advocating for Both the Patient and Family: Communication is the Key   *51*
Guiding: Walking That Difficult Journey   *52*
A Note on Withdrawing Life-Sustaining or Life-Extending Treatment   *53*
Summary   *53*
References and Other Resources   *54*

Chapter 7: After the Death: The Long Journey to the Car   55
What Happens After a Patient Dies?   *55*
Skilled Clinician: Understanding Grief   *55*
Advocating for the Family: Accommodating Their Comfort Needs   *57*
Guiding the Family: Accepting the Loss   *57*
Self Care   *60*
Summary   *60*
References and Other Resources   *60*

Chapter 8: When a Child is Dying: Pediatric End of Life Care   63
Children Die Too   *63*
Skilled Clinician: Assessing and Intervening in the Care of Children   *65*
Advocating for Children: Meeting the Needs of Both the Patient
    and the Family   *66*

Guiding Children and Families: Understanding the Needs of the Child 68
Summary 69
References and Other Resources 69

Chapter 9: Cultural Sensitivity: Looking Through Different Eyes *71*
Making Room for Cultural Diversity *71*
Understand Your Own Beliefs *72*
Listen to the Patients *73*
Avoid Stereotyping and Making Assumptions *74*
Use Trained Medical Interpreters *74*
Use Community Resources *75*
Advocating for Patients and Families *75*
Summary *76*
References and Other Resources *76*

Chapter 10: Hospice: The Gold Standard for End of Life Care *79*
A Philosophy of Care **79**
Who Qualifies for Hospice Care? *80*
How Do I Approach Patients and Families About Hospice Care? *81*
The Hospice Medicare Benefit *81*
Advocating for Your Patients *82*
Summary *83*
References and Other Resources *83*

Chapter 11: A Final Note: Taking Care *85*
Burning Brightly, Burning Dimly *85*
Living in the Present Moment *86*
The Joy and Laughter *86*
A Final Note *87*
References *87*

Index *89*

Foreword

I Didn't Know What I Didn't Know

Twenty years ago, when I was a new, inexperienced home care nurse, I was assigned to Margaret, a 70-year-old woman with terminal liver cancer. She lived with her husband and a disabled son. For five months, I struggled in vain to make her comfortable, to control her pain, to relieve her physical symptoms. I watched her diminish in front of me, her skin breaking down, her eyes glazed with pain, and felt a growing helplessness.

Looking back, I know she sensed my helplessness. I remember walking into her bedroom one day with dread. She was comfortable only in fetal position on her left side. It agonized her to be moved. Her husband's eyes said, "Do something." In desperation, I held her and asked, "Is there something more I can do for you?"

"No," she whispered. I didn't believe her.

Back then, *I didn't know what I didn't know*. I didn't know that her pain and symptoms could be managed, that dying is multilayered and multidimensional, and that Margaret's personal, family, and spiritual suffering could be addressed. I didn't know the crucial role that nursing could have played in helping Margaret die peacefully and comfortably. I wasn't truly present for Margaret or her family.

This book is a primer for nurses in end of life care. It is not meant to be a comprehensive text or an all-inclusive manual. Rather, it is meant to educate nurses enough to *know what you don't know*.

Three Nursing Roles

For many of the chapters, I have divided the nursing role into three parts: the nurse as a skilled clinician, an advocate, and a guide.

Skilled Clinician

This refers to the assessment and technical skills needed to manage care for someone at the end of life. If I'd had the clinical skills to care for Margaret, I would have known how to assess her pain, how to use other health care team members, and how to intervene to keep her comfortable.

Advocate

This refers to the work a nurse needs to do to obtain and assure the best care for a patient. If I'd had advocacy skills, I would have insisted on better pain relief from Margaret's doctor. I would have looked at my home care agency and worked on assuring social work availability for Margaret's family and clear systems for reaching a nurse on call.

Guide

This refers to the knowledge, communication, and intuition a nurse needs in order to walk with a patient during that difficult last journey. If I had been a skilled guide for Margaret, I would have been able to better prepare her for her death. I would have been able to help her husband with simple assurance. I would have been there for her husband and son's walk into bereavement.

This book is written for all the nurses who have the courage and willingness to walk with your patients on that final journey. It is my hope that when you do this, you will be a full witness to the fundamental richness and grace of the human spirit.

Linda Norlander, RN, MS

Where to Begin 1

Death is not a medical event. It is a personal and family story of profound choices, of momentous words, and telling silences.

– Steve Miles, MD

Introduction

Greg is 46 years old. He was diagnosed seven months ago with non-small-cell lung cancer. He has gone through a course of chemotherapy and radiation treatments. His oncologist has just told him that the tumor in his lung is growing and there are few treatment options left. His oncology nurse is part of the conversation. When the doctor leaves, Greg turns to her and asks, "Does this mean I'm dying? What am I supposed to do now?" The nurse sits quietly with him for a few moments—"I want you to know that we will stay with you through this."

Greg has reached a point in his illness where cure is no longer possible. Compassionate and comprehensive nursing care can assure that his needs will be met during his life's final journey. His oncology nurse has begun this care by listening to him and assuring him that he won't be abandoned. One of her next steps will include helping him discuss his care wishes and goals.

Guiding Principles of End of Life Care

While death has remained a constant over the course of history, the process of dying has changed in the last 100 years. Medical advances have taken death from the realm of a sudden event to an often long journey of many events. We have increased the life span, created some complex medical choices, and shaped a new population of people with *chronic illnesses*.

We have not done well, however, in providing care at the end of life. Major reports over the past five years have highlighted nationwide concern regarding health care at the end of life. These reports have chronicled poor pain control and suffering in those who are dying; lack of family inclusion in decision making and care; and inconsistent and conflicting decision making by the health care system (SUPPORT 1995).

Nursing has been on the forefront of many advances in end of life care including pain and symptom management. Yet, nurses continue to enter practice with little or no experience caring for dying patients. A recent review of nursing textbooks discovered that only 2 per cent of the overall content related to end of life care. Equally disturbing, the researchers found that the information was often inaccurate (Ferrell et al. 1999). Even practicing nurses express a discomfort with caring for people who are dying (Last Acts 2000). In order to help patients like Greg, we need to understand what end of life care is all about and be skilled practitioners of nursing arts.

First and foremost, end of life care is patient goal centered and provided for those who have a limited life expectancy. The term "palliative care" is often used when discussing end of life care. Palliative care refers to an intensive program of care with treatment goals to relieve pain and suffering (Lattanzi-Licht et al. 1998).

The best end of life care encompasses a holistic approach that recognizes the physical, personal, family, and spiritual realms of the patient. The patient's family should always be considered as part of the unit of care. Five Guiding Principles for End of Life Care can help nurses frame a comprehensive and compassionate plan for patients and families. (See sidebar, Guiding Principles for Comprehensive End of Life Nursing Care.)

Core Nursing Responsibilities: Skilled Clinician, Advocate, and Guide

Ten years ago 22-year-old Jennifer's father was dying of leukemia in a busy public hospital. She sat with him alone, the only family member at the bedside. The nursing staff avoided his room. Jennifer agonized with every breath her father took, interpreting his gasping as a struggle. Finally, in desperation to give him relief, she took off his oxygen mask. To her horror, her father stopped breathing. She blamed herself for his death. No one sat with her or explained to her what those final moments would look like. She held onto this secret for years until she finally confessed to a friend who was a hospice nurse, "I think I killed my Dad." Her nurse friend assured her that she was not responsible for her father's death and that she gave him a precious gift by being at his side when he died. On hearing this, Jennifer began to cry. "I've carried this all these years. You mean I didn't kill him?"

Years of guilt and suffering for Jennifer could have been averted by a competent and compassionate nurse at the time her father was dying. Jennifer and her father needed a nurse competent in three core ways to care for them through his dying:

- A *skilled clinician* who understood symptom management at end of life and could provide the best comfort care for Jennifer's father.
- An *advocate* who could assure that all members of the health care team were available to Jennifer and her father.
- A *guide* who could walk with Jennifer and her father through the dying experience.

What Do Patients and Families Want for Care at the End of Life?

The first step for a nurse in becoming a skilled clinician, an advocate, and a guide is a clear understanding of what patients and families want for care at the end of life.

Guiding Principles for Comprehensive End of Life Nursing Care

1. Patient and family preference for treatment and care will be discussed and respected. Nurses will:
   - Ask about patient and family goals and preferences
   - Include patient and family in the decision process
   - Provide assistance and resources to formulate advance care plans
   - Honor written health care directives
2. Undesirable symptoms will be relieved. Nurses will:
   - Believe reports of distress
   - Do their best to relieve all undesirable symptoms
   - Anticipate and prevent undesirable symptoms when possible
   - Provide urgent treatment of severe symptoms
3. Emotional, spiritual, and personal suffering will be addressed. Nurses will:
   - Ask about emotional, spiritual, and personal suffering
   - Offer the help of interdisciplinary or community resources
4. Patients will be prepared for their death, and families will be prepared for the death of their loved one. Nurses will:
   - Provide honest information on what is likely to happen
   - Provide guidance in planning how to handle predictable events
5. Grieving will be acknowledged. Nurses will:
   - Provide a quiet and safe place for families to grieve
   - Accommodate family wishes to be with the deceased loved one
   - Acknowledge that grieving is a long-term process

(adapted from recommendations by the Minnesota Commission on End of Life Care 2001)

Studies and surveys have identified that the key desires of patients and families at the end of life are process oriented and relationship based rather than focused on medical goals (Project DECIDE 1996; Steinhauser et al. 2000). They want:

- **Pain and symptom management:** Patients want assurance that physical discomfort will be relieved.
- **Family involvement:** Patients want their families involved in decision making and in care.
- **Care at home:** When asked, most patients express a desire to receive their end of life care at home.
- **Preparation for death:** Patients want to know what will happen as they near death.
- **Completion:** Patients want the opportunity to say good-bye and leave some kind of legacy.
- **Affirmation of the whole person:** Patients want to be recognized as still having something to contribute. They want to be a person first, then a person who is dying.

When Do We Start Providing End of Life Care?

The shift from a focus of curative care to a focus on palliative and end of life care does not usually begin with a sudden event. For most patients who are nearing the end of life, the journey has been long—sometimes years. Patients describe a roller coaster ride with periods of very good times and periods of very low times. Often as they ride the roller coaster, they experience some type of incremental decline. Good palliative and end of life care is often delayed because of the failure to recognize changes in the patient's condition. Look for indicators that signal the need to begin discussions on end of life care. (See sidebar, Red Flags, that can signal the need to begin discussions on end of life care.)

A good nursing assessment involves careful attention to the whole person. Ask these questions:

- Has the patient changed? How was the patient six months ago? Three months ago? Two weeks ago?
  - Lost weight?
  - Less energetic, less able to do everyday activities?
  - Increased symptomology? Dyspnea, fatigue, pain
- Has the family seen a change in the last six months? Three months? Two weeks?

> **"Red Flags"**
>
> Red flags that can signal the need to begin discussions on end of life care (Norlander and McSteen 2000):
>
> ▪ Illnesses or conditions that could be considered potentially life-threatening or life-limiting
> ▪ A *change* in functional status with dependencies in two or more ADLs
> ▪ Repeat hospitalizations and emergency room visits
> ▪ Anyone for whom you would answer "yes" to the question: Would you be surprised if this person was alive in one to two years?

Once a patient has been determined to be at risk for dying, the change from curative to a palliative focus of care still might be gradual. For some patients this shift might never occur. As nurses who advocate for patients and help guide them, it is our responsibility to help facilitate ongoing discussions with the patients about their care wishes and goals. No matter what setting you practice in—hospital, nursing home, clinic, or home—it is of utmost importance that you attend to the patient's comfort needs *as the patient sees them.*

A Team Approach

The needs of patients and families at the end of life are multidimensional. As nurses, you have a large toolbox of skills ranging from clinical and technical skills to assessment and communication skills. However, in caring for dying patients and their families, it's important to recognize that you can't do it all. A good clinician draws on the expertise of other professionals to enhance practice and provide the highest level of care.

For example, a recent study identified dying patients' needs to achieve spiritual peace (Steinhauser et al. 2000). The patient might best accomplish this with assistance from a chaplain, community clergy, or a counselor. Referral to other professional resources may be as important to a patient's comfort as administering the most appropriate dose of morphine. Professional team members to utilize when caring for patients at the end of life can include a wide variety of people.

Physician

The role of the physician in the care of dying patients cannot be overstressed. Not only do physicians direct clinical care, but they have the expertise in disease pathology. Most important, patients and families often look to the physician more than anyone else for guidance during these difficult times.

Social Worker

Social workers are skilled in communication, in group facilitation, and are knowledgeable about community resources. They can be critical in helping patients with long-term planning, in helping to facilitate family discussions, and in counseling patients and families.

Chaplain or Spiritual Care Worker

Many of the issues that patients and families deal with during life's final journey revolve around spiritual and religious matters. Treatment decisions are sometimes based on religious beliefs. This is often a time for self-reflection and contemplation. Patients may need help articulating and thinking through some of the basic questions of life such as "What am I here for?" Often hospital and nursing home chaplains as well as community spiritual leaders can be of help.

Pharmacist

Often a forgotten team member, the pharmacist can be of great value in developing the best pharmacological care plan for the patient.

Dietician

Patients and families often struggle with nutrition and hydration issues. Dieticians can counsel on types of foods to prepare, supplements, and feeding methods.

Other Team Members

Other team members to consider include physical, occupational, and speech therapists, psychologists, volunteers, and clinical nurse specialists. The best nursing care at end of life is provided in a team atmosphere. Beware of feeling like you have to be all things to all patients. Use your resources.

Summary

Comprehensive nursing care for patients at the end of life can only be provided using a holistic approach. The five guiding principles of end of life care can provide a framework for care. Patient and family goals and wishes need to be discussed. Care must be taken to address the physical, personal, family, and spiritual needs of the patient. The best care is provided in an interprofessional team environment. Your nursing role includes being a skilled clinician, advocate, and guide.

References

Ferrell, B., R. Virani, and M. Grant. 1999. Analysis of end-of-life content in nursing textbooks. *Oncology Nursing Forum* 26(5): 869–76.

Last Acts Media Center, May 3, 2000, www.lastacts.org

Lattanzi-Licht, Marcia, Jay Mahoney, and Galen Miller. 1998. *The Hospice Choice.* New York: Fireside Books, p. 44.

Miles, S. 1996. Foreword. In *Hospice Care, A Physician's Guide.* St. Paul: Minnesota Hospice Organization, p. 5.

Minnesota Commission on End of Life Care Report, 2001, www.minnesota-partnership.org

Norlander, L. and K. McSteen. 2000. The kitchen table discussion: A creative way to discuss end-of-life issues. *Home Healthcare Nurse* 18(8):532–539.

Project DECIDE: A roundtable report to the community. 1996. Minneapolis: Allina Foundation.

Steinhauser, K. et al. 2000. In search of a good death: Observations of patient, families and providers. *Annals of Internal Medicine* 132(10):825–832.

SUPPORT Principal Investigators. 1995. A controlled trial to improve care for seriously ill hospitalized patients. *JAMA* 274:1591–1598.

Other Resources

Albom, Mitch. 1997. *Tuesdays with Morrie.* New York: Doubleday.

Lynn, J. and J. Harrold. 1999. *Handbook for Mortals, Guidance for People Facing Serious Illness.* New York: Oxford University Press.

Choices at the End of Life: Advance Care Planning 2

"It's always a little tough to talk about one's own mortality, but I've come to grips with it. After all, I've been at death's door three times now."

— Home care patient discussing advance care planning

The Courageous Conversation

Stephanie is a 62-year-old divorced woman with two children and three grandchildren. Four months ago she was diagnosed with ALS (amyotrophic lateral sclerosis). Since her diagnosis she has experienced increased lower extremity weakness. Three days ago she fell, suffering a soft tissue knee injury and fracturing her right wrist. She is hospitalized for surgery to stabilize the wrist. When the nurse comes in to care for her, Stephanie starts to cry. "How am I going to go home like this? What happens if I get worse? I've heard that some people go on breathing machines. I'm not sure I want that." While the nurse bathes Stephanie she asks, "Have you talked with your doctor about what you might see with this illness?" Stephanie says, "No. I've been waiting for her to bring it up." The nurse sits by the bedside with Stephanie and says, "I'd like to spend a few minutes with you. Can we talk about some of these things?"

Stephanie's nurse is embarking on a difficult and courageous conversation. This talk is the beginning of advance care planning for Stephanie. These discussions are not easy for either the patient and family or the nurse. We live in a society that is not comfortable talking about dying. For example, a recent poll found that people in the baby boom generation (born between 1946 and 1964) are more comfortable talking with their children about safe sex than talking with their terminally ill parents about death (NHF 1999). As nurses, we have not been trained to have these conversations. Yet, too often critical end of life care discussions are delayed until a patient is in crisis or too close to death to participate (Hume 1998). Earlier identification of patient wishes can prevent inappropriate and often unwanted treatments.

Skilled Clinician: *Understanding the Elements of Advance Care Planning*

Clinical nursing skills in working with patients at the end of life include a knowledge and understanding of advance care planning. If you know the key elements in the discussion with a patient and family about end of life care goals, you can facilitate a therapeutic interaction. (See sidebar, Key Elements of Advance Care Planning Discussion.)

Advance care planning is a thoughtful, facilitated discussion that encompasses a lifetime of values, beliefs, and goals for the patient and family. It is not merely a discussion of medical treatment choices. People make decisions throughout life based on their experiences, values, goals, and sociocultural norms. Making decisions about how one would like to be treated at the end of life is no different. Completion of an advance directive (also known as a living will or health care directive) can be part of advance care planning, but this is only one component in a much larger discussion.

People who are significant to the patient, such as family, friends, and caregivers, should be invited to participate in the advance care planning discussion as the patient wishes and allows. However, discussing end of life issues may be a topic that patients and their loved ones, in an effort to protect each other, find difficult to discuss openly. You can be extremely helpful as an objective, skilled clinician to guide these discussions and clarify thoughts and feelings that the patient and family have.

Any advance care planning discussion should be held in a setting that is comfortable for the patient and family. One of the most effective places to have this is in the

---

Key Elements of Advance Care Planning Discussion

Helping a patient and family talk about end of life wishes and goals involves understanding some key elements of the discussion (Norlander and McSteen 2000):

- Patient goals and values
- Patient experience with death
- Patient understanding of illness
- Family support and understanding of patient goals and values
- Communication with physician
- Resources

patient's home. For nurses working in institutional settings, it is not possible to gather a patient and family "around the kitchen table." However, you can strive to make the setting as comfortable and informal as possible. Is it private and free from distraction? Are the chairs comfortable? A cramped examination room, for example, is not the best place for initiating such important and vital communication.

Patient Goals and Values

Advance care planning is an opportunity for a respectful, therapeutic discussion with patients as they think about how they want to die. Patient goals and values are at the heart of any advance care planning discussion. Some patients value living a long life, or living an active life, or enjoying the company of friends. Others place financial concerns as a top priority. Goals can be very broad or very specific. One patient expressed the goal that she wanted to live long enough to see the birth of a grandchild. Another wanted to make sure he could leave a financial legacy for his children. An important question to ask regarding care goals is, "What do you hope for?"

Patients also often have a strong preference for where they would like their care as they are dying. A 72-year-old widower said, "I grew up in this house. I've lived here all my life. This is what I know. I'd like to stay here until I die." As noted in Chapter 1, most people would like to be in their own homes.

Patient Experience with Death

A patient's own experience with the death of a loved one can have a profound impact on care wishes at the end of life. For example, an 85-year-old patient with congestive heart failure expressed a great fear of dying in a nursing home. When the nurse explored this with her, she explained that her husband had died in a nursing home and she didn't want her children to experience that again. A middle-aged man, who had witnessed his father's death when he was a child, expressed a fear of dying in extreme pain. You can ask the question, "What has it been like for others you've known when they died?"

Patient Understanding of Illness

It's important to explore how patients understand the illness. Do they see it as life threatening? Are they expecting a cure or improvement? Do they understand their treatment choices? How a patient views the illness can be very different from how the medical profession sees it or how the family understands it. At the beginning of one advance care planning discussion, a family specifically asked the social worker not to say anything about dying to the patient because he didn't know he was terminal and he might lose hope. To the family's surprise, when the social worker asked the patient his understanding of the illness, the patient said, "Well, it's pretty obvious, isn't it? I'm dying." A way to find out what a patient knows is to say, "Tell me what you know about your illness," or, "What has the doctor told you?"

Family Support of Patient Goals and Values

An effective advance care planning discussion must involve the patient's family. Discuss any conflict or disagreement with a patient's wishes. As one patient stated, "I'm glad we've discussed this because those decisions won't fall on the children now." This is an opportune time to name someone as the health care proxy, the spokesperson if the patient is unable to speak or make decisions.

Physician Communication

Patients look to their physicians for guidance during the course of a disease. You can help patients and families frame the questions to discuss with the doctor. You can also be invaluable in clarifying the patient and family understanding of what the physician has said.

Resources

A discussion of resources available to patients is an integral part of advance care planning. Many patients do not know that they have options that can help, such as hospice, community senior services, and community church support. This is also the opportunity to help a patient fill out a health care directive that will provide written documentation of care wishes. For example, after an advance care planning session, a patient requested extra brochures on hospice. "I'm going to show these to my doctor and tell him this is what I want when it's time."

Advance Directives

Advance directives are legally binding documents that direct health care and decision making when patients are no longer able to speak for themselves. Legislation on the use of advance directives and the form they must take varies from state to state.

Generally, two types of advance directives exist.

- **Living Will or Health Care Directive.** The living will is a document filled out by the patient with specific instructions on health care. It often will address issues such as artificial nutrition and hydration and use of resuscitation and intubation.
- **Durable Health Care Power of Attorney, Health Care Agent, or Health Care Proxy.** With this document patients can designate a specific person to speak for them if they are unable to speak for themselves.

A Note on DNR/DNI Status

Patients and sometimes nurses become confused about the difference between a health care directive and a "DNR/DNI" (do not resuscitate/do not intubate) order. They are not the same. A health care directive is a legal document reflecting the *pa-*

tient's wishes for treatment at the end of life. A DNR/DNI is a *physician's* treatment order. DNR/DNI status written in a patient's chart does not mean an advance care planning discussion has taken place.

Advocating in Advance Care Planning: Making Sure Wishes are Honored

Nurses play a key role not only in initiating and facilitating discussion about end of life care, but in making sure that these wishes are honored. You can advocate for your patients on several levels.

First, on the patient/family level, find out if the patient has an advance directive. If not, offer the resources to facilitate the discussion. Use the skills of other health care team members such as the social worker or chaplain. Engage the physician in the discussion by setting up a time the patient and family can talk with him/her about treatment preferences.

If the patient does have an advance directive, ask the important question, "Does this document reflect your current wishes?" Make sure that the patient and family understand what has been written. Also make sure that the care orders reflect the patient's wishes. A large multihospital study found that even when a written directive was in the chart, only 25 per cent of the physicians were aware they existed. In this study, patients with written advance directives were no more likely than patients without them to have their preferences for or against CPR honored (Covinsky et. al. 2000). Patients and families sometimes assume that if choices are written down, they will be honored.

On an organizational level, ask these questions:

▪ Do you have a system for making sure that advance directives are honored? When a nurse in a Midwestern skilled nursing facility discovered that advance directives were ignored because they were "buried" in the back of the chart, she changed the system to have a listing of treatment wishes placed in the Kardex.

▪ Do you have the professional team support to help if disputes or issues arise regarding patient care wishes? If not, consider forming an interdisciplinary ethics committee.

Guiding in Advance Care Planning: Recognizing the Common Barriers

As discussed earlier, this can be a difficult yet courageous conversation for the patient and family and the nurse. Several challenges exist including how to approach the subject with patients and how to overcome common barriers to the discussion. (See sidebar on Helpful and Supportive Phrases.) Recognizing some of the common barriers to the discussion will help you as you sit down with the patient and family.

Will the Patient Lose Hope If I Bring Up the Topic?

Many nurses fear that if they bring up the subject of end of life care wishes, the patient might lose hope. However, research has shown that the actual process of discussing end of life issues stimulates therapeutic conversations between patients and health care professionals, and it leaves patients and families with an increased sense of feeling cared for and understood (Miles et al. 1996).

The most important need of patients and families is assurance that they will not be abandoned and that every effort will be made to optimize the highest quality of life in their remaining days. With this understanding, you can work with patients and families in determining goals for treatment at the end of life, and the patient and family will be better able to trust that you will continue to support them in any situation.

Isn't Advance Care Planning the Physician's Responsibility?

The physician should be one of the health care team members involved in advance care planning. The physician might know more about prognosis and treatment of a particular diagnosis, but the nurse often has a much better perspective on how a patient is functioning. This is an opportunity for you to prepare patients and families for a discussion with the physician and also empower them to state their care wishes and goals.

I'm Not Comfortable Talking About Death and Dying.

Nurses may find that in talking about advance care planning with patients, their own personal experiences and issues may be brought to the surface. Your own personal history of loss and death can have a positive or negative impact on professional prac-

---

Helpful and Supportive Phrases

Helpful and supportive phrases that could be used to initiate the advance care planning discussion include:

- "Have you thought about what kind of care you would want if you could no longer speak for yourself?"
- "Making decisions before a crisis is a gift you can give to your family."
- "Advance care planning gives you some control over your future."
- "This is an opportunity to develop a written health care directive."

tice. Nurses are encouraged to explore their own feelings, beliefs, and experiences. Completing a health care directive for yourself can be a helpful exercise and improve your comfort level with the process.

Decision Making at the Time of a Crisis

Much as it would be nice to know a patient's care wishes at the end of life, advance care planning is often not done. If you work in an acute care setting, especially an intensive care unit or emergency room, you might be faced with distraught patients and families trying to make hard decisions about such aggressive treatments as resuscitation, intubation, artificial nutrition and hydration, and dialysis. In emotionally charged times such as these, your guidance with good communication and listening skills is essential:

- **Clarify choices in simple language.** Patient and families might not understand the word "intubation" but they should understand "a tube that is placed in the windpipe and connected to a breathing machine."
- **Explore possible preferences with the family if the patient is unable to speak.** If the patient is unable to speak and does not have a health care directive or agent, ask the family if they can recall any conversations with the patient that would indicate the patient's wishes.
- **Clarify "benefit versus burden."** If a treatment is chosen, what are the benefits and what are the burdens associated with it? Will it make the patient more comfortable? Extend life? What kind of care will be involved? What can be expected to happen in two days or two months?
- **Engage other team members.** Often, patient and families find comfort in talking with a chaplain or community clergy before making decisions.

Common Questions Patients Ask About Advance Directives

The advance directive document can be very confusing for patients and families. In the nursing role as a clinician, advocate, and guide, it's helpful to be prepared for some of the common questions patients and families have.

- **I already have a will. Why do I need to fill out one of these forms?** Patients are often confused by the array of legal terminology and become mixed up between the words "will," "living will," "power of attorney," and "health care power of attorney." Reiterate to the patient that a will and a power of attorney refer to financial and estate planning, not health care planning.
- **Do I need a lawyer to help me with an advance directive?** *No.* Advance directives are health care decisions and can be filled out by the patient and family or

with assistance from a nurse, physician, or other health care professional (Sabatino 1998).

- ▪ **Who should I name as my health care agent?** Nurses can help facilitate the decision on who the patient will name as his agent (medical power of attorney or proxy) by asking the patient who he trusts to carry out his wishes. It's important that the patient discuss care wishes and goals with this person before naming them as the proxy.
- ▪ **Will my wishes be honored?** In most states, health care professionals are legally bound to honor the patient's wishes. Sometimes this does not occur for several reasons:
  - ● The advance directive is not available at the time treatment decisions need to be made. This is especially true in emergency situations.
  - ● The advance directive is not clear. Statements such as "no heroic measures" can be interpreted in many different ways.
  - ● The health care proxy is unsure of the patient's wishes.
- ▪ **Can I change my mind?** Every patient has the right to change or revoke an advance directive. In fact, patients often rethink treatment decisions during the course of an illness. Review advance directives with patients on a periodic basis.

Summary

Advance care planning is much more than asking patients if they have a "Living Will" or if they want to be resuscitated. It's a comprehensive and therapeutic discussion of patients' values, care wishes, and goals at the end of life. It is a vital component of holistic nursing practice for any patient with a life-limiting illness.

References

Covinsky, K.E. et al. 2000. Communication and decision-making in seriously ill patients: findings of the support project. *Journal of the American Geriatric Society* 48:S187-S193 (Supplement).

Hume, M. 1998. Improving care at the end of life. *The Quality Letter for Health Care Leaders* 10:6.

Miles, S.H., R. Koepp, and E.P. Weber. 1996. Advance end-of-life treatment planning: A research review. *Archives of Internal Medicine* 156:1062–1068.

National Hospice Foundation (NHF). 1999. Survey, April 9-20. Washington, DC.

Norlander, L. and K. McSteen. 2000. The kitchen table discussion: A creative way to talk about advance care planning. *Home Healthcare Nurse* 18(8):532–539.

Sabatino, C.P. 1998. 10 legal myths about advance medical directives. *ABA Commission on Legal Problems of the Elderly*. American Bar Association: Washington, DC.

Other Resources

Books

Norlander, L. and K. McSteen. 2001. *Choices at the End of Life: Finding Out What Your Parents Want Before It's Too Late.* Minneapolis, MN: Fairview Press.

Websites

1. Aging with Dignity
Website: www.agingwithdignity.org
Provides the health care directive document "Five Wishes," which is legal in 36 states.
2. Caring Conversations: Making Your Wishes Known for End-of-Life Care (A program offered by the Midwest Bioethics Center)
Website: www.midbio.org
Program components include a workbook on end of life issues, a resource booklet of consumer education about health care and end of life decisions, an adult study group guide and video, and other resources.
3. Partnership for Caring, Inc. (previously Choices in Dying)
Website: www.partnershipforcaring.org
1-800-989-9455 (WILL)
Provides a 24-hour hotline offering up-to-date information about advance directive laws for individual states and general information about end of life issues and decision making. Also provides individual states' legally recognized advance directive document.

Pain Management: It's More Than Knowing the Meds 3

Listening to the Patient's Pain

Jackie is in her early forties. Two years ago she was diagnosed with a rare terminal neurological condition. She has gradually lost her ability to control her legs and to walk. As her disease progresses, she is experiencing more pain. She has found, during clinic visits and hospitalizations, that both the doctors and the nurses have been reluctant to address her pain.

"They say to me, 'Oh, you can't be in that much pain,' or, 'We don't want to prescribe too much medication because you might become addicted,' or, 'You just have to live with it. That's part of the disease.'"

She is currently hospitalized with a possible bowel obstruction related to the progression of her disease. During this hospitalization her nurse listens to her story and says, "I believe you are in pain. Let's work with the doctor to make you more comfortable." Jackie begins to cry. "You mean you'll help me?"

Unfortunately, Jackie's story is not unique. Pain is one of the most undertreated conditions in modern medicine. One of the largest scientific studies conducted on care of the dying found that 40 per cent of patients who died in the study were in mild to severe pain at the time of their death (Lynn et al. 1997). For those who are dying, pain represents one of the greatest fears. A 1997 Gallup poll asked, "What worries you when you think about your own death?" Sixty-seven per cent responded that they were worried about great physical pain before dying (Gallup 1997).

The role of the nurse in pain management cannot be overemphasized. As skilled clinicians, we need to be competent in assessing pain and understanding the principles of pain management. As advocates, we need to work with physicians and other health care team members to develop the most effective care plan for the patient. As guides, we need to work with the patient and the family to find the highest level of comfort.

The first step is to understand what pain is. Pain may be defined as "an unpleasant sensory and emotional experience associated with actual or potential tissue damage or described in terms of such damage" (AHCPR 1994, p. 12). More importantly, though, pain is unique to each person and must be defined as *what the patient says it is* (AHCPR 1994, p. 24). It's very important not to make a subjective judgment on a patient's pain. Remember Jackie's experience. "No one would believe me when I said I had pain." (See sidebar, Phrases to Avoid.)

Skilled Clinician: Assessment and Management of Pain

Many hospitals, nursing homes, and home care agencies are starting to look at pain as a crucial part of the ongoing patient assessment. Most of us are very familiar with the four major vital signs: temperature, pulse, respirations, and blood pressure. Pain is being added as the *fifth vital sign* and being assessed on the same schedule.

The first step required in managing pain is to complete a thorough and organized pain assessment. Failure to do so is a common reason for undertreatment of pain. (See sidebar, the ABCs of Pain Assessment.)

A complete assessment of pain includes the following:

▍ **Pain history:** When did the pain begin? What is the current medication regimen?
▍ **Description:** A patient's description of the kind of the pain can help you better assess the most appropriate medication. Words can include dull, aching, gnawing, cramping, shooting, piercing, sharp, or burning.

Phrases to Avoid

▍ He doesn't look like he's in pain.
▍ She couldn't be in pain—it hasn't been four hours since her last medication.
▍ His pain couldn't be *that* bad. The patient in the next bed has a much more serious condition and he isn't complaining.
▍ We don't want you to become addicted.

ABCs of Pain Assessment

Known as the ABCDE of pain assessment and management, the following is a helpful way of looking at how we can approach a patient.

- **A** **Ask** about pain regularly. **Assess** pain systematically.
- **B** **Believe** the patient and family in their reports of pain and what relieves it.
- **C** **Choose** pain control options appropriate for the patient, family, and setting.
- **D** **Deliver** interventions in a timely, logical, coordinated fashion.
- **E** **Empower** patients and their families. **Enable** patients to control their course to the greatest extent possible.

(AHPCR, p. 24)

- **Pain intensity or severity rating:** Most pain intensity ratings are variations of a well validated numerical scale of zero to ten, with zero representing no pain and ten indicating the most severe pain imaginable (Daut et al. 1983).
- Have patients rate their pain using a pain intensity scale that they can most easily understand. Patients should also be encouraged to keep a log of pain intensity scores at home to report during follow-up visits or phone calls.
- **Location:** Ask the patient to indicate exactly where the pain is occurring and if it radiates. Be aware that it is common for patients to have more than one location and type of pain at any given time.
- **Effects on quality of life:** How does the pain affect the patient? Has it impacted relationships? Does it interrupt sleep? Affect appetite? Increase patient's dependence on others?
- **Precipitating factors:** What makes the pain worse? Is it associated with certain activities?
- **Relieving factors:** What helps? Is the pain better at certain times? Be aware that patients and families frequently use home remedies in addition to prescribed pain medications. They are also becoming increasingly knowledgeable about complementary therapies, such as acupuncture and homeopathic preparations, but may be hesitant to share these practices with you. Ask specifically if they have tried any complementary therapies and how they have helped.

A nursing assessment is not complete until you've discussed with the patient and the family the goals of pain control. Do not assume that you know what the patient hopes to achieve—*ask!* Some patients will want to be completely pain free, even if it means that they will be more sedated. Others are willing to put up with a certain level of pain to be mentally clear. As one patient said, "The morphine makes me pretty sleepy. I want to take a little less today so I can be alert when my five-year-old granddaughter comes to the hospital to visit."

Some patients, because of age, language barriers, or cognitive impairment, might not be as able to communicate as well about their pain. It's important to still do as thorough an assessment as possible. Pain might need to be assessed in other ways such as simpler pain assessment tools, picture scales rather than numeric scales, or translated pain assessment tools.

Principles of Clinical Pain Management

The following principles are based on the recommendations of the World Health Organization (WHO 1990):

- Individualize the treatment regimen to the needs of the patient and family caregivers.
- Use the simplest dosage schedule and least invasive pain management modalities first.
- Follow the WHO three-step analgesic ladder:
  - **Step One.** For mild to moderate pain, use a non-opioid, such as ibuprofen or acetaminophen. Consider adjuvant medications.
  - **Step Two.** For persistent or increasing pain, add an opioid. Consider adjuvant medications.
  - **Step Three.** For continuing pain, or for moderate to severe pain, increase the opioid potency or dose. Consider adjuvant medications.
- Medicate on a regular schedule, not a p.r.n. basis, to assure consistency in the blood level of the medication. This will prevent recurrences of pain.
- In addition to the regularly scheduled medications, have "breakthrough" or "rescue" doses of pain medication available as needed. *Remember*—as the regularly scheduled dose is increased, the breakthrough dose must also be increased.

Avoid polypharmacy. The patient should be on only one long-acting opioid for constant pain. The breakthrough drug should be the immediate-release preparation of the sustained-release drug if possible; i.e., a patient taking sustained-release morphine should use liquid morphine for breakthrough rather than an oxycodone or codeine substance.

Important note: One of the most distressing side effects of opioid pain therapy is constipation. The vast majority of patients taking opioids will need to be placed on a regularly scheduled bowel program including laxatives and stool softeners. This is essential in assuring your patient's comfort and avoiding the complications from constipation. Assess and monitor bowel status regularly.

Use of Adjuvant Medications

Adjuvant pain medications enhance the effectiveness of other conventional analgesics and also provide independent analgesia for specific types of pain. It's important to understand the role of adjuvant medications as a part of the patient's complete pain regimen. Listed below are common adjuvants and their uses.

- **Antidepressants** are very effective for neuropathic pain.
- **Anticonvulsants** are also used to manage neuropathic pain, especially pain described as "lancinating" or "burning," or other neuropathic pain that does not respond to antidepressants.
- **Corticosteroids** provide an anti-inflammatory effect and are useful for severe metastatic bone pain and in reducing pain and headaches associated with cerebral and spinal cord edema. They are the first line of defense in the emergency management of increased intracranial pressure and epidural spinal cord compression.
- **Nonsteroidal anti-inflammatory drugs (NSAIDS)** are the first line treatment for bone metastases and other inflammatory conditions.

Complementary or Integrative Therapies

A growing body of research is identifying the therapeutic value of non-pharmacy interventions in pain (Pan et al. 2000; AHCPR 1994). Complementary or integrative therapies are becoming widely accepted by both the lay public and health care professionals. When used to *supplement* the prescribed medication regimen, patients can derive much benefit and comfort from non-drug therapies. In addition, teaching family caregivers complementary therapies that they can easily do to improve the patient's comfort may improve their feelings of being useful and involved in their loved

---

Complementary or Integrative Therapies

Some common complementary approaches to pain management are listed below. Nurses can easily do some of these therapies; others will require referrals to the appropriate therapist.

- Massage Therapy
- Therapeutic Touch
- Physical Therapy: exercise, range of motion, ultrasound
- Heat / Cold Application
- Acupuncture / Acupressure
- Relaxation and imagery / Meditation

---

one's care. (See sidebar for listing of Complementary or Integrative Therapies used for pain relief.)

Advocating: Assuring That the Patient's Pain Relief Goals are Met

When Helen's mother was admitted to a nursing home with a terminal breast cancer, she came under the care of a new physician who did not know her well. Helen could see she was in pain. "I was fortunate because the charge nurse was so helpful. First she figured out that Mom needed to be on pain pills on a regular basis. When that still didn't make her comfortable, she was on the phone right away to the doctor to get stronger medication. When the doctor was reluctant to prescribe morphine, the nurse just kept at him and kept at him until we got what we needed for Mom."

The first rule in advocating for your patient is that pain beyond the patient's expressed goal is *unacceptable.* Achieving the acceptable level of comfort might require clinical skills, persistence, and finesse. Start with a thorough patient pain assessment. Perhaps the solution is as simple as working with the physician to change the pain regime from p.r.n. to regularly scheduled doses.

Communication with the physician is key to advocating for your patient. Be aware that not all physicians are skilled in pain management (AHCPR 1994). However, most care deeply about the needs of their patients. If the physician is struggling with the pain management plan, look for assistance from other team resources. Can the pharmacist help? Does your hospital, nursing home, or clinic have access to pain specialists or a palliative care team? Is a hospice program available for a pain consultation?

Communication with the patient and family is another key to advocating for the best pain management. Patients can also pose problems that interfere with good pain relief. For example, many patients are afraid to take opioids because they fear addiction or constipation. Furthermore, many fear that if they start taking a medication like morphine now, they won't be able to have enough pain relief later (AHCPR 1994). Families often have the same concerns. As a son said, "But Dad, I don't want you to become addicted." It is your role to inform and educate and, above all, to reassure.

The advocacy role does not stop with an initial pain management plan that meets the patient's goals. You need to ask the question, is this plan sustainable? For example, perhaps you have an elderly patient who is on around-the-clock every-four-hour doses of oxycodone while hospitalized. Is it reasonable for the patient to maintain that schedule once he's home? Factors to consider include:

▪ **Future setting for the patient.** Can this plan be maintained at home? In a nursing home? Assisted living? Relative's home? This is an excellent time to consult with other team members such as the social worker.

- **Cost**. Medications can be expensive and not always covered by insurance. Is the route, dose, and brand of medicine the most cost-effective? Is the patient eligible for hospice under Medicare? The Hospice Medicare Benefit covers the cost of pain medication.
- **Cultural considerations**. Make sure the pain management plan is culturally acceptable to the patient and family. In some cultures, the primary decision-maker might be someone other than the patient. If this is the case, the decision-maker must be part of the pain management planning.
- **Environment**. Some opioids have a "street value" for illegal sale. Does the patient live in a high-risk area? If so, patient safety must be a consideration. Can the medication be converted to one with less street value? Consult with the pharmacist on the best way to manage the medication in these circumstances. Also consider that in high-risk areas, local drug stores might not carry the medication.

As an advocate for the best pain management for your patients, it's also essential to look at the system or organization you work in. Do barriers exist that inhibit timely pain relief for your patients? Consider:

- Does your hospital, nursing home, or home care assess pain on a regular basis? If not, what can you do to change the policies?
- How quickly does your system respond to pain management problems? For example, one hospital discovered that it took nearly two hours from the time orders were received on pain management until medication was administered (Lynn et al. 2000). By implementing assessment and response standards, they were able to reduce this to 30 minutes.

Guiding Patients and Families: Addressing Common Myths

One of the most important roles you have as a nurse in working with dying patients is that of a guide. This is particularly true in pain management. By understanding the fears and myths that accompany pain, you can guide and teach patients and families.

Myth: Narcotic Addiction

If I take narcotics, I risk becoming addicted.

One of the greatest fears expressed by patients and families about opioids is that taking them will cause addiction.

Fact

Addiction is defined as a psychological dependence, often resulting in antisocial and destructive behaviors. The literature shows that abuse of therapeutic opioids by patients is rare (Portnoy and Payne 1992). When working with a terminally ill patient, the concern over addiction is irrelevant and harmful in that it interferes with appropriate attention to the comfort and quality of life for the patient.

Myth: Fear of Diminishing Returns

If the pain is worse, then my disease is worse. If I take more medication, it will eventually stop working.

Many patients actually underreport their pain for fear that more pain means the disease is getting worse. Others fear that if they take more medication, it will eventually stop working for them.

Fact

Patients with many chronic conditions live well for years on varying doses of opioids and other pain medications. While increased pain can be a sign that the disease is worsening, it does not foreshadow the end of life. Developing tolerance to opioids is generally slow, and all pure opioids (i.e., not in combination with other non-opioids such as acetaminophen) have no maximum daily dose or "ceiling" on analgesic effect. In other words, pure opioids can be dosed as high as clinically necessary to achieve pain management.

As a guide, listen to your patients' fears and help them weigh the benefits versus burdens of their pain management plan. Actively engage both the patient and the family in the pain management plan. (See sidebar on Engaging the Patient and Family in the Pain Management Plan.)

Know the Resources

One of the best ways you can be effective in managing your patient's pain is to know the resources. Many excellent books and web resources are available that

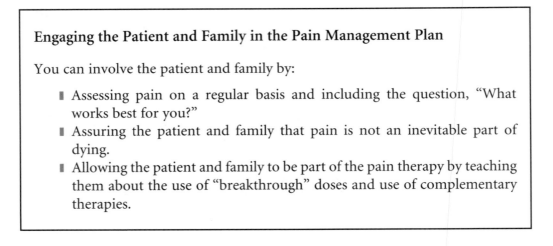

Engaging the Patient and Family in the Pain Management Plan

You can involve the patient and family by:

- Assessing pain on a regular basis and including the question, "What works best for you?"
- Assuring the patient and family that pain is not an inevitable part of dying.
- Allowing the patient and family to be part of the pain therapy by teaching them about the use of "breakthrough" doses and use of complementary therapies.

provide guidelines on types of pain medications, dosages, and use. If you do not have them available to you at your place of work, ask to have them added to the library or resource shelf. See Other Resources at the end of this chapter for some suggestions.

Summary

As a skilled clinician, your first step in managing pain is a thorough assessment. Begin by asking the patient. Know the basics of pain management and use other team resources. As an advocate, be persistent in assuring that your patient's pain is managed. Assess your workplace and work to remove barriers to timely and effective pain management. Consider pain as a fifth vital sign.

As a guide, listen to patient and family fears about pain and pain management. Work with the patient and family to dispel myths about pain. Teach the patient and family how to manage pain using both medications and other therapies.

References

Agency for Health Care Policy and Research (AHCPR). 1994. *Management of Cancer Pain, Clinical Practice Guideline Number 6.* Rockville, MD: U.S. Department of Health and Human Services.

Daut, R.L., C.S. Cleeland, and R.C. Flanery. 1983. Development of the Wisconsin Brief Pain Questionnaire to assess pain in cancer and other diseases. *Pain* 17: 197–210.

George Gallup International Institute. October 1997. Spiritual Beliefs and the Dying Process, Key Findings from A National Survey. Nathan Cummings Foundation and Fetzer Institute.

Lynn, J. et al. 1997. Perceptions by family members of the dying experience of older and seriously ill patients. *Annals of Int. Med.* 126:97-106.

Lynn, J., J.L. Schuster, and A. Kabcenell. 2000. *Improving Care for the End of Life: A Sourcebook for Health Care Managers and Clinicians.* New York: Oxford University Press, p. 41.

Pan, C.X. et al. 2000. Complementary and alternative medicine in the management of pain, dyspnea, and nausea and vomiting near the end of life: A systematic review. *Journal of Pain and Symptom Management* 20(5):374–387.

Portney, R.K. and R. Payne. 1992. Acute and chronic pain. In Lowenison, J.H., P. Ruiz, and R.B. Millman (eds.). *Substance Abuse: A Comprehensive Textbook, 2nd ed.* Baltimore: Williams and Wilkins, pp. 691–721.

World Health Organization (WHO). 1990. Cancer pain relief and palliative care. Report of a WHO expert committee. Geneva, Switzerland: WHO, pp. 1–75.

Other Resources

Books

Ferrell, B.R. and N. Coyle (eds.). 2001. *Textbook of Palliative Nursing.* New York: Oxford University Press.

McCaffery, M. and A. Beebe. 1989. *Pain: Clinical Manual for Nursing Practice.* St. Louis: C.V. Mosby.

McKay, Peter. 1998. *Symptom Control in Hospice and Palliative Care.* Essex, CT: Hospice Education Institute.

Wrede-Seaman, L. 1999. *Symptom Management Algorithms: A Handbook for Palliative Care.* Yakima, WA: Intellicard.

Websites

1. www.edc.org.painlink

PainLink is a virtual community of health professionals working in institutions that are committed to alleviating pain.

2. www.eperc.mcw.edu

End of Life Physician Education Resource Center (EPERC) has information and links on a variety of topics related to end of life care.

3. www.growthhouse.org

Provides resources and links to other websites.

4. www.lastacts.org

Provides up to date information on management of care at the end of life and links to other organizations.

Physical Symptom Management: Knowing What to Look For 4

Sometimes he would close his eyes and try to draw the air up into his mouth and nostrils and it seemed as if he were trying to lift an anchor.

– Tuesdays with Morrie (p. 153)

Common Symptoms

Edgar is a 68-year-old man with end-stage congestive heart failure. He has been hospitalized three times in the last six months for a variety of problems. He has just been transferred to a skilled nursing facility following a hospitalization for pneumonia. The transfer document indicates a very poor prognosis. When the admitting nurse sees him, he appears to be restless and uncomfortable. However, when she asks him to rate his pain, he says he has none. The nurse then says, "You seem to be so uncomfortable. Can you tell me about it?" Edgar tells her that sometimes he feels like he can't catch his breath. "I'm afraid I'm going to suffocate and you won't know what to do." The nurse says, "Let's see about having some medication on hand in case you feel like you're having trouble breathing." She talks with the doctor and arranges for oxygen and liquid morphine to control his dyspnea.

When patients are dying, many distressing physical symptoms may be present that need to be assessed and addressed. While management of pain is of utmost importance, we also need to pay careful attention to a wide array of other problems that can cause a patient great discomfort. (See sidebar, Common Symptoms Associated with Patients at the End of Life.)

> **Common Symptoms Associated With Patients at the End of Life**
>
> - Dyspnea
> - Constipation
> - Diarrhea
> - Nausea
> - Weight loss and loss of appetite (anorexia and cachexia)
> - Skin disorders
> - Asthenia and fatigue
> - Anxiety
> - Depression

Skilled Clinician: Assessment and Management of Common Symptoms

The first step in alleviating the discomfort from these symptoms is a thorough assessment. The assessment includes a medical history and a history of any current symptoms. Questions to ask:

- "Tell me about your health. What is the history of your illness?"
- "Tell me about your most distressing symptoms."
- "Are you having any problems with nausea, constipation, breathlessness, poor appetite, etc?"
- "What helps these symptoms? What doesn't help?"

A complete symptom assessment also looks into functional status and how symptoms have affected the patient's activities of daily living and relationships. Remember from Chapter 1—a patient at the end of life wants to be affirmed as a "whole" person. Assessment questions include:

- "Has/have your symptom/s affected your ability to be independent?"
- "Has/have your symptom/s affected your family or loved ones?"
- "Have you experienced changes in your routines because of your symptom(s)?"

These questions can get to the heart of what's causing the discomfort for the patient. For example, a patient who was having difficulty with urinary frequency was less concerned about the physical problem than he was about the burden it placed on his wife, particularly at night. The nurse established a plan in the hospital that included reducing fluids in the evening and arranging for a bedside commode to be sent home with the patient at discharge.

In approaching and assessing symptoms, keep in mind that above all you are looking for the *patient's* perception of the problem. Families sometimes report symptoms or ask for symptom relief for problems that are more distressing to them than to the patient. If a family member says, "Do something. He looks so miserable," it's important to ask the patient, "Is this a problem for you?"

Clinical approaches to some of the common symptoms can involve pharmacology as well as basic comfort techniques and complementary therapies.

Dyspnea

It is estimated that between 29 and 74 per cent of dying patients experience difficulty breathing (Lynn et al. 1997). Breathlessness can be one of the most distressing symptoms for both patients and their families. First look at the cause. For example, treatment for dyspnea associated with congestive heart failure might include diuretics to relieve fluid build up. Treatment for dyspnea associated with anxiety might include antianxiety medications. Common palliative approaches to dyspnea include:

- **Oxygen and humidified oxygen via nasal prongs.** Nasal prongs can be irritating to the skin and nostrils. Monitor the skin regularly for signs of irritation.
- **Opioids.** Opioids can be a very effective treatment for dyspnea. It is believed that they work by altering the central perception of dyspnea much in the same way they alter the central perception of pain (Farncombe and Chater 1993).
- **Inhalers and nebulizers.** Saline nebulizers or inhalers with beclomethasone or albuterol used on a regular basis can provide relief. Nebulized morphine can also be an effective and relatively noninvasive way to relieve dyspnea.
- **Anxiolytics.** Breathlessness can be exacerbated by anxiety. A wicked cycle can occur if a patient feels panic because of the dyspnea. Anxiolytics can be used in conjunction with other therapies to relieve the symptoms.

Dyspnea relief can also be achieved without the use of pharmaceutical intervention. (See sidebar, Simple Remedies to Relieve Breathlessness.) In addition, comple-

---

Simple Remedies to Relieve Breathlessness

- Using a fan to help circulate the air
- Opening a window
- Restricting the number of people in the room
- Repositioning the patient by elevating the head of the bed

---

mentary therapies can be used. Acupuncture, acupressure, and progressive relaxation have shown some efficacy in relieving breathlessness (Pan et al. 2000).

Constipation

About half of dying patients experience some form of constipation due to a variety of factors including use of opioids for pain relief, decreased mobility, and decreased appetite (Muir et al. 1999). The foremost clinical goal in addressing constipation should be that of prevention. This means assessment of bowel status should be routine, particularly for those patients receiving any type of opioid treatment including mild opioids such as codeine. It's also important in assessing for constipation to ask the patient, "What are your common bowel habits?" Therapy can then be adjusted to fit the patient's needs. (See sidebar, Common Treatments for Constipation.)

Dietary and other interventions can also be effective for some types of constipation. Prune juice, for example, works as a stimulant laxative. In putting together a bowel program, ask the patient, "What works best for you?" One patient, when asked, said, "Every morning I retire to the bathroom with the crossword puzzle. It's worked for me for years. But here in the nursing home, I can't do that anymore."

Diarrhea

While diarrhea is a less common symptom for patients in the terminal stages of illness, it can be both disruptive and dehumanizing (Muir et al. 1999). It can be caused by a variety of underlying conditions including bowel obstruction, medications, gastrointestinal bleeding, and poor absorption. Common treatments include use of antidiarrheal medications and, in some cases, fluid replacement. Dietary interventions should also be considered, such as avoidance of gas-producing foods and lactose.

Common Treatments for Constipation

- **Stimulant laxatives.** These work by stimulating bowel activity. Common ones include senna, casanthranol, and bisacodyl.
- **Osmotic laxatives.** This type of laxative draws water into the bowel. They include lactulose, milk of magnesia, and magnesium citrate.
- **Stool softeners.** These increase the water content of the stool. They include sodium docusate and calcium docusate. A combination of laxative and stool softener is often the most effective for patients taking opioids.
- **Lubricant stimulants and enemas.** Therapies in this category range from glycerin suppositories to soap suds enemas.

(EPEC Project 1999, Module 10)

Nausea and Vomiting

Close to 60 per cent of terminally ill patients experience some type of nausea. Thirty per cent experience vomiting (Muir et al.1999). Nausea and vomiting in patients can be caused by a variety of problems ranging from increased cerebral pressure to mechanical obstruction, medications, or infections. Clinical treatment for nausea and vomiting varies depending on the underlying cause. Fortunately, studies have shown that distressing symptoms can be controlled in over 90 per cent of patients.

Weight Loss and Loss of Appetite

Perhaps one of the most disturbing symptoms for a family to see is the weight loss and loss of appetite in a loved one. We associate nourishment closely with love. When assessing this symptom, find out how the patient feels. Often the patient is far less disturbed by inability to eat or by the weight loss than the family is. Pharmacologic interventions can include megestrol, prednisone, or dexamethasone to stimulate the appetite and control other symptoms such as nausea and vomiting (Storey 1996). Nonpharmacologic interventions include:

- Offering the patient favorite foods and nutritional supplements.
- Reducing portion sizes and eliminating dietary restrictions.
- Discussing with the patient and family together the natural progression of the disease and what alternatives can be used in place of food to show love and nurturing.
- Using alcohol such as a glass of wine as an appetite stimulant. (Of course, first assess for a history of alcohol-related chemical dependency.)

Skin Disorders

The skin is the largest organ in the human body. Because of disease pathology, nutrition, hydration, and mobility issues, terminally ill patients are particularly vulnerable to skin problems. Prevention of skin disorders such as pressure sores is the first line of defense. However, sometimes even the most meticulous care will not stop skin breakdown or discomfort. Common types of skin problems include:

- **Pressure ulcers.** Palliative goals should focus on prevention of further breakdown, and management of discomfort and odor (Bates-Jensen et al. 2001). Pay particular attention to the heels, sacrum, and elbows. Interventions include frequent turning and repositioning, as well as use of specialized pressure-reducing surfaces such as mattress overlays or low-air-loss beds. Meticulous hygiene and positioning is also essential.
- **Pruritus and skin irritation.** Skin itching and discomfort can be a source of great distress for patients. First start with a thorough assessment including location and description of the discomfort—itching, burning, tickling, "pins and needles." Depending on the type of discomfort, interventions may include

thorough cleansing, warm baths, cold packs, and topical creams. Sometimes systemic pharmaceuticals such as corticosteroids, antidepressants, or antihistamines are needed to provide relief (Rhiner and Slatkin 2001).

Fatigue

Loss of energy and tiredness is normal in the progression of a terminal condition. This does not make it any less distressing for the patient or the family. Often helping the patient and family to understand the progression of the disease and to adapt to the patient's fluctuating energy level can be effective. Patients can also suffer from boredom and understimulation due to inactivity. Encouraging the patient's favorite activities even in a modified form can be very restoring (Dean and Anderson 2001). You can also enlist the assistance from other health care team members such as the physical therapist or occupational therapist to suggest ways of assisting the patient to conserve energy. Pharmacological interventions include the use of steroids or low-dose stimulants.

Anxiety

A multitude of issues can trigger feelings of anxiety in a patient who is facing the end of life. Fear of the future, worry about loved ones, fear of pain, and a general feeling of being overwhelmed by all that is happening can cause patients to be distressed. Anxiety can be seen several ways in patients including increased agitation and restlessness, breathlessness, hyperventilation, and profuse sweating. Pharmacologic treatments include use of medications such as benzodiazapines. Careful assessment and use of the interdisciplinary team can be key to relieving anxiety. (See Chapter 5 on suffering.)

Depression

About 50 per cent of terminally ill patients experience some type of depression (Muir et al. 1999). By recognizing and managing depression, you can make it possible for the patient and family to not only experience personal growth together, but complete life closure (EPEC Module 6 1999). Depression can be characterized by persistent feelings of hopelessness and helplessness. Depressed patients express feelings of despair and worthlessness such as "What good am I to anyone anymore?" Depression is also linked to a vicious cycle with pain for the patient—the more pain the more depressed, and the more depressed the more pain. (See sidebar, Questions to Ask Patients About Depression.)

The first step in treating depression is to address the distressing physical symptoms such as pain. The second step is to engage other team members including the physician, social worker, or psychologist to create a comprehensive treatment plan. Depression in terminally ill patients can be treated with antidepressant medications, counseling, and alternative therapies such as relaxation and guided imagery. Assess and intervene as early as possible. Patients often don't have the time left that it takes for some interventions, particularly pharmacological-based therapies, to take effect.

In cases of a very short prognosis, low-dose amphetamines can be helpful in lifting the mood. Remember also, not all terminally ill patients are depressed. It's important to distinguish between depression and normal life-closure behavior. For example, a patient can express concern about being a burden to the family without being depressed (Block 2000).

Advocating: Linking the Needs of the Patient and Family to the Medical System

As an advocate, you are the link between the needs of the patient and family and the medical system. You need to make sure that the patient receives a comprehensive symptom assessment and that the identified needs of your patient and family are addressed. This means not only charting the assessment but following through to achieve a comprehensive care plan. The most expertly done and written assessment is of no use if it's filed away at the back of the chart. For your patient this might mean:

■ Direct and immediate discussion with the patient's physician regarding assessed needs
■ Recommendations for other disciplines such as social work, chaplain, dietician, or therapist to be involved
■ "Watchdogging" orders through the system. It is not acceptable for a patient to be in distress for hours because of a bureaucratic system.

Keep the plan of care patient and family centered. For example, if it's important to the patient to have family members at the bedside, can you change restrictive visiting hours to accommodate this? On the other hand, if the patient is in distress because of too much company, intervene on the patient's behalf. Even small things can make a difference during this difficult time. The wife of a dying patient said, "Even though my husband could not eat, it was important to him that I get my meals. The nurse always ordered a tray and brought it for me. We felt like the hospital really cared."

Know and use the resources available to you. Does your health care center have a palliative care nurse specialist or consult service? Do you have access to hospice care? One of the richest and most comprehensive resources available to patients and families at the end of life is hospice care. Hospice care is available to patients in their place of residence whether that's home, a nursing home, or some other type of facility. Consider asking the physician for a referral to hospice. (See Chapter 10, Hospice Care.)

Guiding Patients and Families: Preparing, Listening, and Assuring

Our nursing role as guides for patients and families can ensure comfort and symptom management. As noted in Chapter 1, patients and families want not only comfort but preparation for the dying experience. As a guide you can:

- **Assure patients that their symptom needs will be addressed.** For example, you can say, "I know that nausea and upset stomach are distressful for you. We are going to try a new medication. If that doesn't work, we have some other therapies. Here's what you can expect when we start the medication…"
- **Explain therapies in terms patients and families can understand.** Instead of saying, "We're going to start oxygen at 2 liters per nasal cannula," try, "Sometimes a little extra oxygen can help you breathe better. We're going to start some oxygen that will come through this tube directly into your nose. It will make a little whooshing noise. That way, you know it's on. If it makes you uncomfortable let us know."
- **Prepare patients and families for what might come next.** "You should find with this new medication that you will be sleepy at first, but once you get used to it, that side effect will go away. It usually takes a day or two."
- **Listen carefully to what the patient and family say about symptoms.** If a patient says, "I get this real anxious feeling at night when the lights are turned off," you might want to offer to leave the lights on, the curtain open, or the door open.
- **Engage the patient and family in the care plan.** Teach the family how to turn and position the patient for more comfort. Ask, "What would you like to know? What are your goals?"

In whatever way you can, always give a clear message to the patient and the family that you will not abandon them.

Summary

One of the guiding principles of nursing care at the end of life is relief of undesirable symptoms. As a skilled clinician, you need to know how to assess and intervene with a variety of physical symptoms. As an advocate, you need to make sure that problems are addressed in a timely manner, that the resources of the team are used, and that your system is hospitable to both the patient and family. As a guide, you need to begin preparing the patient and family for death and to engage them as much as possible in the care giving and decision making.

References

Albom, M. 1997. *Tuesdays With Morrie.* New York: Doubleday.

Bates-Jensen, B.M., L. Early, and S. Seaman. 2001. Skin Disorders. In Ferrell, B.R. and N. Coyle (eds.). *Textbook of Palliative Nursing.* New York: Oxford University Press.

Block, S.D. 2000. Assessing and managing depression in the terminally ill patient. *Annals of Internal Medicine* 132:209-218.

Dean, G.E. and P.R. Anderson. 2001. Fatigue. In Ferrell, B.R. and N. Coyle (eds.). *Textbook of Palliative Nursing.* New York: Oxford University Press.

EPEC Project. 1999. American Medical Association. Module 6 and Module 10. www.ama-assn.org

Farncombe, M. and S. Chater. 1993. Case studies outlining use of nebulized morphine for patients with end-stage chronic lung and cardiac disease. *Journal of Pain and Symptom Mangement* 8:4; 221-225.

Lynn, J. et al. 1997. Perceptions by family members of the dying experience of older and seriously ill patients. *Annals of Internal Medicine* 126: 97-106.

Muir J.C. et al. 1999. Symptom control in hospice—state of the art. *The Hospice Journal* 14:33-61.

Pan, C.X. et al. 2000. Complementary and alternative medicine in the management of pain, dyspnea, and nausea and vomiting near the end of life: A systematic review. *Journal of Pain and Symptom Management* 20(5): 374-387.

Rhiner, M. and N.E. Slatkin. 2001. Pruritus, fever and sweats. In Ferrell, B.R. and N. Coyle (eds.). *Textbook of Palliative Nursing.* New York: Oxford University Press.

Storey, P. 1996. *Primer of Palliative Care.* Gainesville, FL: American Academy of Hospice and Palliative Medicine.

Other Resources

Doyle, D., G.W.C. Hanks, and N. MacDonald. 1998. *Oxford Textbook of Palliative Medicine.* Oxford, England: Oxford University Press.

Kaye, Peter. 1998. *Notes on Symptom Control in Hospice and Palliative Care.* Essex, CT: Hospice Education Institute.

Suffering: It's Not Just the Pain 5

Until I did the assessment, neither the patient nor I realized that her distress was not due to her pain, but to her suffering.

– Hospice Nurse

What is Suffering at the End of Life?

Mrs. S. is an 80-year-old woman with ovarian cancer living alone in her own home. A home care nurse sees her on a weekly basis. During the visits, the nurse observes that Mrs. S. is restless and unable to sit for long periods of time before she needs to get up and pace. The home care nurse has asked her on several occasions if she is in pain. Mrs. S. always says, "No." Several medications have been prescribed to help "calm her down." Nothing appears to work. During today's visit, the nurse says, "I'm concerned because you seem so uncomfortable. Is something else going on?" Mrs. S. starts to cry and says, "I'm afraid to die."

Comfort for a patient doesn't always mean physical symptom relief. In order to address patients' comfort, we must also address their suffering. In his groundbreaking work on suffering, Dr. Eric Cassel defined suffering as "a state of severe distress associated with events that threaten the intactness of the person" (Cassel 1991). The first step in intervening in a patient's suffering is to understand that suffering is multidimensional and sometimes difficult for a patient to articulate. For nurses who care for dying patients, suffering needs to be looked at in terms of its physical, personal, family, and spiritual aspects.

The second step in intervening in a patient's suffering is to do a thorough assessment. Ask patients to rate both their pain and their suffering using a 0 to 10 numeric intensity scale. Beyond asking for a rating, ask the key question, "Do you want help in this area?" While many patients acknowledge that they are suffering, not all feel they need intervention (Baines and Norlander 2000). (See sidebar, Key Concepts of Suffering at the End of Life.)

Skilled Clinician: Assessing Suffering

Nursing clinical skills in the area of suffering are linked with understanding the concept of suffering, conducting a thorough assessment, and knowing the resources for intervention. Suffering, like pain, should be based on patient report. Like pain, it's very important not only to ask, but to *believe* the patient's response.

Physical Suffering

Not all physical suffering is due to pain, and not all pain is identified by the patient as physical suffering (Baines and Norlander 2000; Chapman and Gavrin 1993). Physical suffering can be very closely related to issues of quality of life such as independence and self-worth. For example, a patient with ALS rated his pain very low, but when asked about physical suffering, rated it very high: "I can no longer raise my hand to my mouth. Do you understand how humiliating it is to not be able to feed yourself anymore?" Another patient rated her physical suffering as very high because she said, "No matter what I try, I'm cold all the time. I hate to get out of bed." Other sources of physical suffering can include:

Physical discomfort that patients don't identify as pain such as aching, pressure, spasms, cramping, numbness, or tingling.

- Discomfort or distress from immobility. One patient stated, "I can't get out of bed any more and my bones ache."
- Sleeplessness
- Chills or fever
- Declining functional ability and increasing dependence on others. "I used to be able to walk around the block; now I can't walk to the bathroom without resting."

Key Concepts of Suffering at the End of Life

- Suffering is more than pain. It's multidimensional involving physical, psychosocial, and spiritual aspects.
- Suffering can and should be assessed on a routine basis.
- Not all suffering needs intervention.
- Many interventions for patient suffering are within the nursing skill set.
- Those interventions not within the nursing realm can often be performed by other team professionals.

- Appearance changes such as weight loss, loss of hair, disfiguration
- Skin problems such as itching, inflammation, or wounds
- Odors from wounds

Once the source of physical suffering is identified, a plan of care can be devised based on the patient's needs. Interventions vary according to the type of distress. For example, if the patient is miserable because of skin itching, medication or regular use of lotions and creams might be appropriate. If a patient is in distress because of tiredness or weakness, you might consider consulting a physical or occupational therapist to look at ways to conserve patient energy. Or if the patient has identified suffering due to increased dependence on the family for caregiving, you might consider consulting with the social worker on arranging more help for the patient once discharged to home.

Personal and Family Suffering

Personal and family distress can have a wide range of implications. Suffering in this area can be due to relationships, unfinished business, grief, or fears of the future. Some patients have difficulty expressing themselves in this area. Questions to ask might include:

- *How much are you suffering due to loss of enjoyment of life?* A patient with COPD said, "Golf was everything to me. Now I can't play anymore and I sit here day after day just thinking about being outside."
- *How much are you suffering due to your feelings and relationships with family and friends?* A hospice nurse visited a dying patient at home for the first time. She said, "The patient was in terrible pain. Yet, when I asked her about what she wanted, she told me the most important thing to her was not relieving the pain, it was reconciling with her daughter. The first thing I did was arrange for the daughter to come over with a social worker present."
- *How much are you suffering due to your concern for your loved ones?* A patient who rated his suffering high in this area said, "My wife doesn't even know how to write a check. What's going to happen when I'm gone?"
- *How much are you suffering due to fear of the future?* When asked this question, an elderly patient replied, "I'm afraid those doctors are going to do things to me to try to keep me alive. I don't want to be a vegetable in a nursing home."
- *How much are you suffering due to unfinished business?* A young mother told the nurse, "I want to leave something for my daughters to remember me by. But I'm so sick now I can't think what to do for them."

Suffering in the psychosocial realm encompasses a lifetime of beliefs and relationships. With your daily workload you might not have enough time with patients to adequately address all these issues. However, one of the most important clinical skills you can offer to patients is the ability to listen and acknowledge the distress. As

Ira Byock, MD, said, "The optimal way to know the experience of another person is to ask" (Byock 1996, p. 243). You also have the powerful ability to offer the resources of other professional team members including social workers, therapists, and chaplains.

Spiritual Suffering Spiritual Suffering

Perhaps one of the most difficult areas to assess, yet one of the most important for patients at the end of life, is the realm of spirituality. Some have also identified this as existential suffering (Cherny et al. 1994). Others have called it the search for meaning, for hope, or for connections with oneself, others, or a higher power (Corr et al. 2000). Spirituality extends beyond religion and faith beliefs and into the realm of the meaning of life.

A middle-aged woman expressed the complexity of this concept when she recalled her mother's death when she was 16. "A few weeks before she died, Mom looked at me with such anguish in her eyes and asked, 'What was it all about?' She wouldn't live to see me grow up, to see her grandchildren and to realize some of her own dreams. At 16, I didn't know what to say to her. At 50, I still don't know the answer." For assessing a patient in this realm, helpful questions can include:

- *How much are you suffering related to your ability to interact with your spiritual (or faith or religious) tradition?* An elderly homebound man expressed a high degree of suffering in this area because he'd regularly attended church in his community and received communion. Now that he couldn't get out of the house, he missed his weekly communion.
- *How much are you suffering related to your ability to find strength in your belief system?* Patients might respond to this question with statements about feeling abandoned by their higher power.
- *How much are you suffering related to your feelings about your personal source of inner strength?* This question can bring up feelings of hopelessness or inadequacy. "I used to think I was the strong one in the family, but I'm no good anymore."

Nursing intervention in the area of spiritual suffering begins with listening and acknowledging the distress. You cannot provide meaning for another, but you can encourage patients to tell their own stories. You can also ask, "Would you like help in this area?" Again, remember you can offer the resources of the other professionals on your health care team.

Advocating for Patients: Assuring a Holistic View

Because assessing patient suffering at the end of life can be complex and extends well beyond some of the daily tasks of nursing, it's easy to fall into the pattern of looking only at physical symptoms and needs. As an advocate for the patient and the family, you are critical in seeing that the patient is viewed holistically. On a patient/family level this means addressing suffering as a routine part of your comprehensive patient comfort assessment. Just as you ask a patient, "Can you rate your pain on a 0 to 10 scale?" you can also ask, "Can you rate your physical, personal, family, and spiritual suffering on a 0 to 10 scale?"

As an advocate, be prepared to look for ways to honor your patient's wishes. Patient suffering can be increased by confinement in an unfamiliar bed in an unfamiliar room. Many patients at the end of life want to spend their final time in the comfort of their own home. Consider what you can do to facilitate a discharge to home:

- Advocate for a hospice or home care referral.
- Teach the patient and family the necessary cares before discharge.
- Simplify the medication regime (IV to oral, short-acting opioids to sustained release opioids).

If care at home is not possible, what can you do to make your hospital or nursing home more home like? The first place to start in accommodating the patient and family is to ask them, "What could we do to make you more comfortable?"

Within your health care institution—hospital, nursing home, home care agency, or clinic—you can also advocate for routine suffering and comfort assessments for patients who are dying. Be prepared, however, to meet some resistance. One of the great fears in addressing patient suffering is that you will ask the question, the patient will answer, and you will not know how to intervene. Remember when asking yourself whether you are prepared to address patient suffering:

- Listening and acknowledging patient suffering can be an intervention in itself.
- Not all patients want or need intervention in suffering.
- Many interventions are already part of your nursing skill set, such as active listening.
- You have other interdisciplinary team members who can help.

Guiding Patients and Families: Start with Yourself

For patients who are suffering at the end of life, your skills as a guide are crucial. As you ask yourself, "What can I do to help guide this patient and this family?," remember that the first place to start is with yourself. How comfortable are you caring for a dying patient? A new graduate nurse recalled her first experience with a dying patient. "I did my cares for him as quickly as possible and got out of the room. I could see in his eyes that he was suffering, but I was so afraid he might die while I was with him and I wouldn't know what to do." Your fears and uncertainty can be communicated to the patient and to the family in many ways.

If you are not comfortable caring for someone who is dying, ask yourself why. If you can answer that question, you can grow into your nursing practice.

- *I've never done this before.* You will face death at some time in your career, either professionally or personally. Read up on nursing care for those who are dying. Attend professional education seminars. Talk with your colleagues.
- *I'm afraid I'll do something wrong.* Remember, you are not alone in caring for the patient. You have other professionals. Use them. And use your listening skills. Patients at the end of life need to tell their story. Families need to be heard.
- *What if the patient has a problem I can't fix?* Not all symptoms, suffering, or distress at the end of life can be "fixed." The message to convey to patient and families is, "I will not abandon you, and I will do everything in my power to make things more comfortable."

As a guide to the patient and family, you need to be *present* for them. A nurse who efficiently bathes a patient, changes a dressing, or administers a medication is not necessarily *present*. Presence means listening, touching, acknowledging, and honoring a patient's wishes.

Listening

Listening to a dying patient can be both verbal and nonverbal. You can guide the patient who wants to talk by using open-ended questions such as "Can you tell me more?" Or you can use affirming statements such as, "That must be hard for you." Sometimes sitting silently with a patient can be the most effective form of listening.

Acknowledging

Patients who are at the end of life's journey state they want to be acknowledged as still having something to contribute (Steinhauser et al. 2000). Guidance can include encouraging patients to tell or write their life stories and experiences. This can be done on audio or videotape, through the creation of an ethical will, or through letters. For example, with the encouragement and assistance from a nurse, a young woman dying from breast cancer wrote letters to both her young daughters to be opened on their birthdays each year until they were 18.

Touching

Sometimes families are afraid to touch their loved one for fear they might "disconnect" something such as an IV or a monitor. You can guide families through example and by teaching them simple tasks such as turning, positioning, and massage. You can also guide through your own example. Sit, when talking with the patient. Provide gentle touch as is comfortable for the patient.

Honoring the Patient's Wishes

Patient wishes near the end of life are varied. The first step in honoring those wishes is to simply ask, "What would you like?" One home care patient, when asked what he would really like to have, answered, "A lobster tail." With the encouragement of the nurse who assured the family that at this point in the illness a low fat, low salt diet was not necessary, the family prepared a lobster dinner. While the patient ate very little of it, he loved the festiveness of the occasion.

Summary

One of the guiding principles of nursing care at the end of life is addressing patient suffering. As the nurse for a dying patient, you are in the most powerful position to intervene with suffering. Clinical skills include the ability to assess suffering, intervene where appropriate, and refer to other professional team members. As an advocate, you can work with your institution to make sure that suffering at the end of life is routinely assessed and that barriers to a patient's comfort are removed. As a guide, you can be *present* for the patient and family, acknowledge their suffering, and listen to their needs.

References

Baines, B. and L. Norlander. 2000. The relationship of pain and suffering in a hospice population. *The American Journal of Hospice and Palliative Care* 17(5): 319-326.

Byock, I.R. 1996. The nature of suffering and the nature of opportunity at the end of life. *Clinics in Geriatric Medicine* 12(2): 237-252.

Cassel, E.J. 1991. *The Nature of Suffering.* New York: Oxford University Press, p. 33.

Chapman, C.R. and J. Gavrin. 1993. Suffering and its relationship to pain. *Journal of Palliative Care* 9: 5-13.

Cherny, N.I., N. Coyle, and K.M. Foley. 1994. Suffering in the advanced cancer patient: a definition and taxonomy. *Journal of Palliative Care* 10(2): 57-70.

Corr, C.A., C.M. Nabe, and D.M. Corr. 2000. *Death and Dying, Life and Living.* Belmont, CA: Wadsworth/Thomson Learning.

Steinhauser, K. et al. 2000. In search of a good death: Observations of patients, families and providers. *Annals of Internal Medicine* 132(10): 825-832.

Other Resources

Baines, B. 1999. *The Ethical Will Resource Kit.* Minneapolis: Josaba Inc. www.ethicalwill.com

Ferrell, B.R. and N. Coyle (eds.). 2001. *Textbook of Palliative Nursing.* New York: Oxford University Press.

Active Dying: The Final Days and Hours 6

Wally gave us a gift in the last week of his life: the opportunity to gather as a family, to laugh, to tell stories, and to say good-bye.

— Daughter-in-law of a hospitalized patient

Active Dying: What Does It Mean?

Mrs. N. is an 87-year-old widow who suffered a massive CVA five days ago. No improvement has been noted after several days of active treatment. Mrs. N.'s family has made the decision to forego further treatment including the placement of a feeding tube. Two days ago the IV hydration was discontinued. Mrs. N. is no longer responding to verbal stimulation. Her breathing is labored. The family has been keeping a bedside vigil and is becoming more anxious. They ask the nurse caring for Mrs. N., "Is there something more we should be doing? She seems to be struggling to breathe." The nurse replies, "What you are seeing with her breathing is a normal part of the body slowing down. I'd like to talk with you more about what you can expect to see as she changes."

Nurses who work regularly with dying patients often refer to the final phase of life as the period of active dying. This is the time when physiological and mental changes signal that the patient's bodily functions are shutting down. For the patient and family, this can be a momentous time of completion. It is of utmost importance to include the patient and family in the decision making and care. What happens in those last days and hours can leave a lasting impression on those who live on.

Skilled Clinician: Assessing and Intervening When Death is Near

In order to treat some of the symptoms associated with active dying, you must first understand, then assess, what is occurring in the dying patient's body. Several clinical indicators can signal that death is close. (See sidebar, Clinical Indicators that Death is Near.)

Increased Fatigue and Weakness

As patients near death, their strength and tolerance for activity decreases. Sometimes this is a very gradual process over a period of months or weeks and sometimes it is quite sudden, with changes happening over a period of days. As patients become weaker and are more likely to be confined to bed, nursing care needs to focus on both patient and family comfort.

- For the bed-bound patient, frequent turning, repositioning, and meticulous skin care is essential. This is the opportunity to engage the family in caregiving by teaching positioning and skin care.
- For the family, a clear explanation of what is happening can help alleviate their anxiety. Be prepared to explain in simple terms that the weakness is due to the body "giving out," not the patient "giving up."

Decreased Food and Fluid Intake

One of the most distressing aspects of dying for families is to see a loved one stop eating and drinking. We associate food and fluid with the essence of life. Fears expressed by families include, "But if he doesn't eat, he'll starve," "If he's not drinking, won't he feel thirsty?" Most patients, on the other hand, do not express feelings of either hunger or thirst (Printz 1992). You can help by:

- Listening to the family concerns and providing information about decreased food and fluid intake as part of a natural process. For families who ask about hydration, many studies have shown that it can actually increase patient dis-

---

Clinical Indicators that Death Is Near

- Increased fatigue and weakness
- Decreased food and fluid intake
- Breathing changes
- Skin color changes
- Decreased levels of consciousness
- Other signs
  - Loss of sphincter control
  - Grimacing and involuntary body jerks
  - Inability to close eyes

---

comfort in the last days of life (EPEC Module 12 1999; Kaye 1998). (See sidebar, Discomfort with Hydration.)

▪ Encouraging family members to use alternative care. For example, teach the family how to provide mouth care. Encourage the family to provide comfort to the patient through touch, music, conversation, or gentle massage.

Breathing Changes

The patient who is dying often does not experience distress as breathing patterns change. However, the family can view the changes as indications that the patient is in discomfort. For example, a pattern of change to very rapid breathing is normal. The family might ask if the patient is feeling air hunger or is suffocating. Common changes as death nears include:

▪ **Periods of very rapid breathing interspersed with periods of very slow breathing.** Use of oxygen does not appear to be of either help or hindrance.

▪ **Periods of apnea.** Patients might breathe normally, then stop for short periods of time, then resume normal breathing. Families describe trying to "breathe for the patient" during the periods of apnea.

▪ **Congestion or gurgling noises.** Perhaps one of the most upsetting aspects of active dying for families is the gurgling sound associated with secretions accumulating in the upper part of the patient's respiratory track. Suctioning is not recommended because it often cannot reach the secretions and because it causes distress to the patient. One of the best ways to treat this is frequent repositioning of the patient and restriction of fluids. Drugs such as scopolamine or atropine that dry secretions can also be helpful. If a patient is receiving IV hydration and respirations are becoming noisy, this might be a good time to discuss with the family discontinuing fluids.

▪ **Agonal breathing.** Agonal breathing has been described as a shallow, pursing of the lips like a fish out of water. This type of breathing is generally what is seen just before a patient dies. It signals that death is near.

Skin and Color Changes

As the body slows down, so does the circulation of the blood. Skin in the extremities can turn a mottled bluish color. Often this is first noted in the feet, hands, and knees. The mottling can progress up the body. Along with color changes, extremities will begin to cool. This can be particularly distressing to families who will ask, "Is he cold? Should we use more blankets?" Provide assurances that this is an expected part of this stage of dying and that the patient is in no distress.

Changes in Levels of Consciousness, Confusion, and Delirium

Patients who are close to dying will often sleep more deeply and become less and less arousable. They might moan or jerk in their sleep. When awake, they might be very clear or very confused. Sometimes they might say things that make no sense to the family. It's not unusual for patients to talk about doors or windows or even maps. Some call this symbolic language or "nearing death awareness" (Callanan and Kelley 1992). Prepare the family for some of these common changes:

- **Confusion.** Patients will often arouse confused about time or place. In addition, they sometimes describe seeing people in the room who have died before them such as a parent or spouse. Assure the family that this is normal, and acknowledge the patient by saying, "I don't see what you are seeing. Are you comfortable?" Reorient the patient to person, time, and place as necessary.
- **Terminal delirium.** Sometimes a patient who has been quiet, even unresponsive, will have a brief burst of energy. It can take the form of restlessness or agitation. Some have described this as heralding "the difficult road to death" (EPEC Module 12 1999). When this happens, families will often mistake this behavior for pain. Increased pain medication generally is not effective. Benzodiazapenes administered orally or buccally have been effective in calming such patients. Again, assure the family and prepare them for this.

Other Signs

Other signs can be present that a patient is nearing death:

- **Loss of sphincter control.** The patient can become incontinent of urine and stool. Pay careful attention to keeping the patient clean and dry.
- **Decreased urine output or inability to urinate.** As the kidneys shut down, urine output decreases. However, do not assume that decreased urine output automatically means kidney failure. As the body slows down, sometimes patients lose the ability to urinate independently. Palpate for a full bladder and observe for signs of agitation or pain. Urinary catheter placement might be necessary.
- **Moaning, grimacing, and involuntary body jerks.** Changes in the central nervous system can lead to these symptoms. Patients can also demonstrate a

"picking" behavior where it appears they are picking at objects floating in the air. The best management for these symptoms is to prepare the family and assure them that they do not indicate that the patient is uncomfortable.

■ **Inability to close eyes.** For families, it can be very distressing to see their loved one with eyes only partially closed and the whites exposed. This happens because of tissue wasting around the eye and eyelid. Use lubricating eyedrops as needed to keep the patient comfortable.

Patients die in their own unique way. Not all signs will be present. When preparing the family for this final stage, explain in brief and simple terms what they might expect, and assure them that you will not abandon them.

A Note on Pain

Little evidence exists that pain increases as a patient nears death. Continue to assess and treat for pain. Continue regularly scheduled pain medications. However, be careful not to overtreat by mistaking some of the common neurological symptoms such as grimacing or moaning as signs of increased discomfort from pain. If you have pain management concerns, this is a good time to consult with another team member such as the physician, pharmacist, or palliative care nurse to determine the best course.

Advocating for Both the Patient and Family: Communicating is the Key

As death nears, you might find yourself in conflicting roles as an advocate for both the patient and the family. These are very highly charged emotional times for the family, and often they will look to you to "do something." In a moment of panic, they might ask for resuscitation, IV fluids, dialysis, or other aggressive measures, even if the patient has clearly stated wishes to the contrary. Communication skills are key here, along with the use of the other team members. If the patient is actively dying and the family wants a change from comfort to aggressive care, your response should be, "Let's involve the doctor and talk about this as a family." Often times, the family needs reassurance that there are no "last ditch" measures that will keep the patient alive. This might also be the time to call in the chaplain or community clergy to talk with the family.

The last phase of dying can be a crucial time for families. It is a time to tell stories and a time to say good-bye. As an advocate for the patient and family, consider what you can do to facilitate an intimate and comfortable environment. If you are in a hospital or nursing home setting, can the patient be transferred to a private room? What can be done to provide more space for the family? Can you arrange for space for the family to bring in favorite photos or mementos?

Families often have little experience caring for or being with someone who is dying. Do you have written resources available to them that will help prepare them for what will come? If not, advocate that your institution or agency add these materials as part of patient education.

Clinically, this is a time to assess the treatments the patient is receiving. Many treatments and procedures that are routine may no longer be necessary and actually cause the patient discomfort (Brody et al. 1997). Look at:

- Daily lab tests
- Frequent assessment of vital signs
- Routine weights
- Any procedure that does not promote the comfort of the patient

Guiding: Walking That Difficult Journey

As a guide, the patient and family are looking to you to walk with them through a very difficult time. In order to do this, you must be confident and competent in understanding what happens during the final days and hours of life. You must be able to communicate well to the patient and family in terms they can understand. Avoid using highly technical terms such as terminal delirium, dyspnea, Cheyne-Stokes breathing, or neurological dysfunction. The phrase "active dying" can also be confusing for the family. (See sidebar, Phrases to Use.)

Families often need guidance at the bedside when the patient is near death and will sometimes ask the question, "What should we be doing?" Suggestions include:

- Assign caregiving tasks, such as mouth and skin care, to family members.
- Teach the family how to do simple complementary therapies such as hand massage.

Phrases to Use

These might include:

- His breathing is changing. He might stop for a few seconds, then start again. This is normal, and it's not uncomfortable for him.
- Often patients will see people from their past. This does not mean that he is "out of his head." We don't know why it happens, but it seems to provide great comfort for the patient.
- It's not unusual to see the blood pressure drop or the heart speed up. This is part of the body slowing down. It is not uncomfortable for her.

- Offer the services of the chaplain, or offer to contact someone from their faith community. Patients and families often find comfort in religious ritual as death nears.
- Suggest the use of music. Note, however, that music is a very personal preference. Do not tune into a music station or play music on a cassette or CD player without the input of the patient or the family.
- Encourage the family to tell stories. Remember, even if patients appear to be unresponsive, we truly do not know what they can hear. Model for the family talking to the patient rather than talking "over" the patient.
- Encourage the family to perform comfortable family rituals such as singing favorite songs, reading passages from the Bible or a favorite book, or reciting familiar prayers.
- Guide the family in saying good-bye. Families sometimes need suggestions of words to use. Consider simple phrases such as "I love you," "I'll miss you," and "Good-bye."

Perhaps the most important role you can play as a guide is to assure the family that there is no right way and no wrong way to do this. Their presence is one of the greatest gifts a family can give to a dying patient.

A Note on Withdrawing Life-Sustaining or Life-Extending Treatment

Nurses working in critical care units are sometimes faced with the emotional and clinical complexities surrounding the withdrawal of life-sustaining treatments. This often includes discontinuing mechanical ventilation, dialysis, and artificial nutrition and hydration. It is of utmost importance during these situations to attend to the comfort of the patient and the needs of the family (Brody et al. 1997). Know the resources available to ensure the best palliation of symptoms during the withdrawal process, and use the expertise of other team members including the pharmacist, chaplain, and social worker. (See M. Campbell, *Forgoing Life-Sustaining Treatment*, under Other Resources.)

Summary

One of the guiding principles of nursing care at the end of life is preparing the patient and family for death. As a patient is dying, nurses need to have strong clinical skills to assess and intervene with some of the symptoms associated with active dying. Communication skills are important to explain to the patient and family what is happening and what to expect. Advocacy includes making sure that families have a safe and comfortable place to be with the patient and that unnecessary treatments and procedures are discontinued. Perhaps one of the most important nursing interventions at this time is the guidance provided to patients and families around communication, rituals, and life "completion."

References

Brody, H. et al. 1997. Withdrawing intensive life-sustaining treatment—recommendations for compassionate clinical management. *The New England Journal of Medicine* 336(9): 652-657.

Callanan, Maggie and Patricia Kelley. 1992. *Final Gifts: Understanding the Special Awareness, Needs, and Communications of the Dying.* New York: Bantam Books.

EPEC Module 12. 1999. American Medical Association.

Kaye, Peter. 1998. *Symptom Control in Hospice and Palliative Care.* Essex, CT: Hospice Education Institute.

Printz, L.A. 1992. Terminal dehydration, a compassionate treatment. *Archives of Internal Medicine* 152: 697-700.

Other Resources

Campbell, M. 1998. *Forgoing Life-Sustaining Therapy.* Aliso Viejo, CA: American Association of Critical Care Nurses.

Ferrell, B.R. and N. Coyle (eds.). 2001. *Textbook of Palliative Nursing.* New York: Oxford University Press.

Karnes, B. *Gone From My Sight.* 1995. Stillwell, KS: Barbara Karnes.

After the Death: The Long Journey to the Car 7

The longest walk in the world is from the room where you have left your loved one, or watched them leave with the funeral home, to the car that is now taking you to an emptier house.

– Reverend Chuck Meyer *(Meyer 2000)*

What Happens After a Patient Dies?

Mr. F., a 69-year-old married man with a history of heart problems, was admitted to the coronary care unit following a massive heart attack. After several days of treatment, he arrested, and attempts to restart his heart were unsuccessful. His wife and two daughters sit numbly in the waiting room as the doctor explains what happened. Recognizing their state of shock and distress, Mr. F.'s nurse asks, "Would you like to be with your husband for awhile?" She and another nurse quickly clean up the room and remove equipment. She brings the family in, makes sure they are comfortable, then asks, "Is there anyone you'd like me to call?"

When a death occurs, nurses continue to be responsible for the well-being of both the patient and the family. Well-being of the patient includes respect for the body and the person the body represents. Well-being of the family means respect and understanding of their grief.

Skilled Clinician: Understanding Grief

Grief is defined as the normal psychological reaction to loss (Kaye 1998). It can be manifested in a variety of ways emotionally, psychologically, and physically. For someone who has experienced an immediate loss, you might see a variety of reactions including sadness, anger, anxiety, confusion, or numbness. Family members might also experience physical reactions such as weakness, dry mouth, or shortness of breath (Worden 1991).

Your communication skills are vital to the clinical management of grief following the death of a patient. How you respond to the family can leave a lasting impression on them. If the death was expected and the family was able to be at the bedside, your first intervention should be a sincere and sympathetic acknowledgement of the death: "I am sorry for your loss."

If the death was unexpected or sudden, it's key that you provide a quiet, comfortable place to talk with the family. It is *inappropriate* to talk with a family about a death in a public waiting room or corridor. Sit down when you talk with the family. Use a preparation phrase such as, "I'm sorry, the news is not good." Explain in simple, nontechnical terms; stop and let the family talk (EPEC Module 2 1999). (See sidebar, Nursing Interventions After the Death.)

Families might feel emotionally numb or simply lost. Ask concrete questions. Rather than saying, "Can I do anything for you?," try, "Can I get you a glass of water?," "Do you have someone I can call for you?," or "Would it be all right if I called the chaplain?"

If you are unable to stay with the family, provide assurance that you are available to them. You might want to set some definite times with them, such as "I'll be back in 15 minutes. If you need me sooner, you can turn on the call light."

If a family member is having a particularly difficult time and manifesting serious physical symptoms such as chest pains or shortness of breath, involve the physician for assessment and treatment. This is also a time when other professional team members such as the chaplain or social worker might provide comfort and assistance.

Sometimes immediate grief might manifest itself in the form of anger or accusations: "Why didn't you do more for him?" Acknowledge the anger and listen in a nonjudgmental way.

Families will also have questions about what to do next. Areas where questions can arise include:

- Organ donation
- Autopsy
- Arrangements for the body and for the funeral

Nursing Interventions After the Death

- Allow the family time to be with the body.
- Observe the family for signs of distress that warrant intervention.
- Listen actively. Often families need to tell their stories.

Know your institution's policies and procedures regarding these areas.

As a skilled clinician, it's also important to recognize that grief is an ongoing process. The patients you are caring for might also be grieving a loss. Their families might have multiple loss issues. Acknowledge those losses and listen with compassion when your patients and families talk about them.

Advocating For the Family: Accommodating Their Comfort Needs

Advocating for the family after the death can take several forms. First and foremost is to provide a quiet, comfortable place for the family. (See above.) If you work in a hospital or nursing home, find space away from public waiting rooms and corridors. Facilitate private, quiet time for the family to spend with the body. Families should not be rushed during this time. For some, this will be the last time they see their loved one. This is a time to say "good-bye."

Respect cultural beliefs and preferences. As much as possible, accommodate the family's needs. This might range from specific rituals at the bedside, to family involvement in washing and clothing the body before it is removed from the room.

Provide professional resources for the family. If they have questions about the medical treatment, arrange for them to spend time with the physician. Facilitate access to chaplains and social workers.

Whether you practice nursing in a hospital, clinic, nursing home, or home setting, bereavement follow-up needs to be a part of any patient plan of care. Work within your system to assure that written resources are available to the family. Some hospitals and institutions have prepared pamphlets that answer some of the immediate questions following a death such as how to handle organ donation, autopsies, funeral arrangements, and death certificates. Every death needs to be acknowledged in some form. Unfortunately, for many families whose loved one has died in an institution, the only contact they have after the death is with the billing department. (See sidebar, Suggestions for Your Health Care Institution or Agency.)

Guiding the Family: Accepting the Loss

Often your nursing involvement following the death of the patient will be short term. However, it's still important to understand what the family will face as they mourn the loss of a loved one. Normal grieving involves four tasks (Worden 1991):

1. Accepting the reality of the loss
2. Working through the pain
3. Adjusting to a life without the loved one
4. Moving on with life

> **Suggestions for Your Health Care Institution or Agency**
>
> - Send a sympathy card to the family. Cards should be culturally sensitive—i.e., without a strong religious message.
> - Provide mailed bereavement follow-up materials such as information on grief groups.
> - Keep a bedside journal where the professional staff can write a note about the patient. This journal can then be sent home with the family.

As you guide the family through the initial loss, you can be especially helpful in the area of accepting the reality of the loss. Acceptance often begins at the bedside while the patient is dying. Encourage the family to be with the patient. As one daughter said, "We sat around Dad's bed, chatting to each other and to him. Suddenly, as a family we *knew* he was about to leave us. No one said anything, we just *knew*. We stopped talking and held hands and were with him when he slid gently away. I wouldn't give those moments up for anything."

Acceptance of the loss comes easier if the family has the opportunity to see the body and to touch it. Ask the family members if they would like to prepare the body in any way. Some will find comfort in providing that last bath. For families who do not want to participate in the preparation, remove equipment, lines, and clutter from the room.

If you are providing nursing care in a hospital, nursing home, or other institution, do not forget "the long walk to the car." When the family is ready to leave, offer to accompany them to the car. Your *presence* sends the message that their loved one had meaning to those who provided care before the death.

In guiding families, be sure you avoid the pitfalls of using clichéd and misguided phrases. (See sidebar, Clichés and Misguided Phrases.)

Children and Loss

Grieving families might look to you for guidance regarding children. Children have three main questions when it comes to a death (Worden 1996)

- Did I cause the death?
- Is it going to happen to me?
- Who is going to take care of me?

Children should have the death explained in a straightforward manner. Avoid using euphemisms such as, "Grandpa has gone to sleep," or "We lost Uncle Bill today." Younger children especially will wonder why no one is trying to wake up

Clichés and Misguided Phrases

"Be Strong" Clichés
- You must be strong for your children.
- You've got to get a hold of yourself.
- Don't cry.

Instead say:
- It's okay to cry.
- I'm so sorry.
- Would you mind if I sat with you for a few minutes?

Religious Clichés
- She's happy with God now.
- It's a blessing.
- God never gives us more than we can handle.

Take your cues from the family and remember that their belief system may not be the same as yours.

Discounting Clichés
- I know just how you feel.
- Be glad you don't have problems like …
- At least you had 30 years together.

Instead use phrases such as:
- He sounds like he was a very special person.
- Let me sit with you for a while.
- Tell me how *you* are doing.

Grandpa or find Uncle Bill. Encourage families to use simple explanations such as "Grandpa died because he was very sick and his heart stopped beating."

In this time of great stress, children will especially need to feel safe and cared for. Observe how the family is responding to any children present. If you are sensing disorganization among the family, you might help direct them by suggesting that one family member be designated to watch over the children.

Reassure families that children should be included in the grieving process as much as the child wants. Children and teens benefit from death rituals and traditions in the same way adults do (Myers et al. 1999).

- Seeing the body reinforces the reality of the death.
- Participating in rituals provides personal meaning.
- Gathering family together lessens isolation.

Self Care

Remember that nurses grieve too when patients die. Allow yourself time to honor the patient who has died and the work you did to care for that patient. A hospice nurse said of her own grief, "I cry with the family. I also try to take some quiet time— sometimes it's a short walk, sometimes I just sit in my car. But I need the time to remember that patient."

Just as families need to share the stories of their loved one, you may need to share stories with other staff. If you work in an institution or agency where you experience a lot of death, consider organizing a periodic memorial service to remember those you have cared for.

Summary

A guiding principle of nursing care at the end of life is the acknowledgement of grief. As a skilled clinician you need to assess and intervene in family grieving. Provide a safe and comfortable place for the family to hear the news of the loss. Allow the family to be with the deceased. Acknowledge the death and recognize that grief is an ongoing process. As an advocate, make sure your institution has procedures in place to acknowledge the death in a caring and compassionate manner. As a guide, be *present* for the family. Listen to their stories and their concerns. Be aware of the special needs of grieving children. Last, but not least, acknowledge your own grief at the loss of a patient.

References

EPEC Project. 1999. American Medical Association. Module 2. www.ama-assn.org

Kaye, Peter. 1998. *Symptom Control in Hospice and Palliative Care.* Essex, CT: Hospice Education Institute.

Meyer, C. 2000. In *On Our Own Terms: Moyers on Dying.* New York: Thirteen/WNET, p. 6.

Myers, R.N., L. Norlander, and J. Young. 1999. *Some Things You May Need to Know When a Loved One Dies.* Minneapolis, MN: Allina Health System.

Worden, J.W. 1991. *Grief Counseling and Grief Therapy: A Handbook for the Mental Health Practitioner, 2nd Edition.* New York: Springer.

———. 1996. *Children and Grief: When a Parent Dies.* New York: Guilford.

Other Resources

Books

Corr, Charles A., Clyde M. Nabe, and Donna M. Corr. 2000. *Death and Dying, Life and Living.* Belmont, CA: Wadsworth/Thomson Learning.

Doka, Kenneth J. and Joyce Davidson (eds.). 1998. *Living with Grief.* Washington, DC: Hospice Foundation of America.

Ferrell, B.R. and N. Coyle (eds.). 2001. *Textbook of Palliative Nursing.* New York: Oxford University Press.

Website

www.growthhouse.org
Provides a listing of books on bereavement and links to other information.

When a Child is Dying: Pediatric End of Life Care 8

A circle no matter how small is still complete.

– Inscription on tombstone for Megan Zaihida Williams 8/26/1991–12/13/1991

Children Die Too

Mark is a 14-year-old male with cystic fibrosis. He is currently hospitalized with a lung infection that is not responding to antibiotics. He has experienced a significant decline in the past six months with increased shortness of breath, fatigue, and weight loss. His mother has asked that no one talk with him about dying. One morning he asks his nurse, "Why won't anyone talk about how I want the rest of my life to go? I know I don't have much time left." The nurse stops what she is doing and sits down at the bedside. She asks, "What would you like to have happen?"

Children are our symbol of life and hope. For children like Mark, dying is complicated by the fact that we believe in a certain order—children should grow up to have families, prosper, and live to be old. Medically, we treat children very aggressively to extend life. On a personal and family level, we are often not honest with children. Caring for children like Mark is one of the biggest challenges nurses can face. (See sidebar, Differences Between Adult Care and Care of Dying Children.)

Nursing competence in caring for children begins with the understanding that, first and foremost, your patient is a child. Second, you are caring for a child who is dying. Caring for a child means understanding needs at different stages of development (Faulkner 1993; Gibbons 1993).

Infants and Toddlers

Children in this age category are learning to be separate from their primary care-givers. They particularly fear abandonment and separation. It's important to provide close and physical contact and minimize separation from parents or primary caregivers. At this age, the concept of death is similar to that of temporary abandonment: "If I die, I'll come back tomorrow."

Preschoolers

Children are developing a sense of initiative. They fear loss of control, bodily injury, and being left alone. Around the concept of death they have fantasy reasoning and magical thinking. Children in this age category often feel a great deal of guilt and responsibility for things they cannot explain. "If I'd washed my hands like Mom said, Grandpa wouldn't have died." Simple concrete explanations are important.

School Age

At this stage, children begin developing logical thought and problem-solving ability. School-age children fear loss of control, failure to live up to expectations of others, and death. They need to have their bodies treated with respect, be offered specific factual information, and have as much control over a situation as possible.

Adolescents

Children at this age are striving for their own sense of identity. They fear loss of control, altered body image, and separation from their peer group. They need honesty and the ability to make as many choices as possible.

With all children, good nursing skills equate with good communication skills. Three questions are important to ask (Doka 1996).

▌ What does the child need to know?
▌ What does the child want to know?
▌ What does the child understand?

Skilled Clinician: Assessing and Intervening in the Care of Children

Assessment of pain and symptoms in children is often complicated by communications difficulties and willingness to participate. Take into account the child's age and developmental stage. For example, most children over the age of four are capable of self reporting pain (McGrath 1990). However, language must be used tailored to the child's own vocabulary. For the child, pain might be called an "owie" or a "hurt."

Often a dual assessment, one person asking the child and one asking the parents, can be helpful. For example, ask the child, "Do you tell others when you hurt?" Ask the parents, "Does your child tell others when he/she is hurting?"

Keep in mind when doing an assessment that children are easily distracted and often times do not appear to be in distress. In one case, the parents reported that their child was not in pain because "he's sitting so quietly watching television." When the nurse explored this further, she discovered that he sat quietly because it hurt so much to move (Hilden et al. 2000).

Sometimes children will underreport a symptom because they are afraid of the treatment. For example, a five-year-old refused to take his morphine tablets. The doctor used the child's favorite teddy bear to talk with the child. She discovered that the child refused the morphine because the tablets were too hard to swallow. She convinced the child to try liquid morphine because it might make his teddy bear feel better (Faulkner 1997).

Children are more likely to talk about what is hurting or bothering them if they feel comfortable with the person who is talking to them. (See sidebar, Tips for Talking With Children About Symptoms.)

Pain

Treating pain in children is similar to treating pain in adults. The analgesic pain ladder from Chapter 3 should be used, beginning with mild analgesics such as acetaminophen and progressing to opioids. The preferred route of administration is oral. Often children will have a permanent IV access, and parents are comfortable with giving meds through an IV. In these cases this route may be the best for both ease and pain relief. Most children do not like the rectal route.

Tips for Talking With Children About Symptoms

- Using language the child understands
- Using play techniques such as puppets or art
- Listening carefully to the child
- Taking your time with the child

Other Common Symptoms

Dying children experience the same array of distressing symptoms as adults. Symptoms include constipation, nausea and vomiting, anxiety, and sleep disturbances.

Anxiety is common in dying children. The first step in approaching this symptom is to make sure that it is not caused by untreated pain. Providing reassurance and emotional support to both the child and the parents are often the most effective therapeutic approaches (Miser and Miser 1993).

Sleep disturbance can be particularly problematic because it is distressing for the child and exhausting for the parent. Drugs such as diphenhydramine, chloral hydrate, or diazepam can be effective (Martinson 1995).

Active Dying

When death is near, your care involves preparing the family for what to expect. The dying process is similar to that of an adult. Common signs to look for include:

- **Alertness and sleep changes.** You may see confusion, restlessness, and a decreased level of consciousness. Encourage the family to maintain gentle physical contact.
- **Breathing changes.** As in adults, breathing may become very rapid, very shallow, and may include 10–30-second periods of no breathing. Sometimes oxygen can be comforting. Also encourage the family to elevate the head of the bed. Assure the family that any gurgling sounds due to secretions are not causing the child discomfort.
- **Temperature changes.** As the heat regulating system fails, the hands and feet can become cool. As in an adult, the child does not usually feel cold with this. You might also see an elevated temperature. Treat with cool washcloths.

Advocating for Children: Meeting the Needs of Both the Patient and the Family

Because the issues in caring for dying children are so multidimensional and complex, the nursing role as an advocate is critical in making sure that the needs of both the child and the family are met.

Communications between Child and Family

One of the most difficult areas to address is communication between the child and the family. As mentioned earlier, a dying child and his or her parents might not be in agreement with the course of care or treatment. Parents are often very protective and reluctant to talk openly with their child about the prognosis. Research has indicated, however, that children are very aware of their prognosis and want to be involved in the decision making. Much of the research done on communication with the dying child shows that families rarely regret sharing too much information but do regret sharing too little (Faulkner 1993).

In advocating for clear communication between parent and child, use the resources of the health care team. If you assess the need, engage the physician, social worker, or chaplain. Many children's programs employ Child Life staff who are trained to address the psychosocial needs of children at different developmental stages. They can also be a helpful resource.

In advocating for communication between the child and the family, also remember that the family includes siblings. Brothers and sisters can often feel left out during the strain and anxiety of a life-threatening illness. They should be included in family conferences and communications as much as possible. Again, Child Life specialists can be of particular help in dealing with sibling issues.

Communications with the Parents

The serious illness of a child places enormous stress on parents. Studies indicate that the better informed parents are about their child's condition, the better they are able to participate meaningfully in care decisions (Hinds et al. 2001). Nursing advocacy includes keeping parents well informed while also assessing their ability to understand and comprehend the information. For example, the mother of a child with a brain tumor said, "Our nurse was incredibly helpful. She gave us information in terms we could understand. Sometimes, when we were overwhelmed, she'd say, 'I'm going to give you some time to absorb all this, then I'm coming back so we can talk again.'"

Effective communications with parents also means taking into account parents in nontraditional families. If the mother and father are divorced, for example, it's important to make sure everyone is informed. Use the skills of other team members such as social workers or chaplains to help facilitate communications in difficult family situations.

Communications With the Doctor

Communication with the doctor is crucial for the patient/family and the rest of the health care team in dealing with a dying child. Researchers have found this to be a problem area. Parents who have lost a child often report that physician communication was vague and confusing. In addition, a survey of pediatric oncologists indicated that 47 per cent do not initiate conversations about advance care planning, but instead wait for families to bring up the topic (Hilden et al. 2001).

Ways to advocate for clearer communications include:

▪ Setting up family conferences that include the physician and other team members
▪ Advocating for communication between physician specialists. In one example, the nurse set up a telephone conference call between the family pediatrician, the pediatric oncologist, and the pediatric cardiologist to make sure the family was receiving a consistent message.

■ Clarifying in simple terminology the level of understanding the patient/family have during a conference with the physician. Asking the question, "Can you tell me in your own words what Dr. X is saying about the chemotherapy?"

Sometimes families don't know what information to ask for. Advocating can also mean helping the family frame the questions for the physician. (See sidebar, What Questions to Ask.)

Care at Home

Studies have shown that most terminally ill children and their families do better when the child is cared for at home (Lauer et al. 1989). As an advocate, especially for a hospitalized child, it's important to ask the question not only of the physician, but of the patient and family: "Can my patient go home?" If the answer is "yes," then you need to follow up with the health care team to make this possible. Make sure you know the community resources for home care and hospice for children.

Guiding Children and Families: Understanding the Needs of the Child

As a guide for your patient and for the family, model the behavior that shows an understanding of the needs of the child. Dying children need (NHPCO 2000):

■ **Love, security, and reassurance**. You can provide this through touch, play, and above all a willingness to listen to what the child says.
■ **Honesty and information**. Communicate in terms of the child's world of understanding.
■ **Control**. Even small choices such as what to eat or which color of medicine to take first can be important.
■ **Privacy**. Children need time to be alone.

What Questions to Ask

■ How will the treatment help my child?
■ What harm might we expect?
■ What will you do with the information if we put our child through another test?
■ Will it change the course of treatment?

■ **Acknowledgement of purpose in life**. Like adults, children want to leave a legacy. This might come in the form of artwork, audio or video tapes, or written work.

In your role as guide, you need to stay with the family even if they make choices or take treatment paths you do not personally agree with. Parents have to make the ultimate difficult decisions about their children. They are the ones who will live on with those choices. It's important to support them in doing what they feel is right.

Summary

Caring for a dying child is one of the most challenging roles a nurse can play. It requires an understanding of the developmental stage of the patient, the unique physiological needs of a growing child, and the complex needs of the family. Advocacy involves promoting communication between the patient, family, and health care system. Guiding means knowing the needs of the patient and being present and supportive for the family.

References

Doka, K.J. 1996. The cruel paradox: Children who are living with life-threatening illnesses. In Corr, C.A. and D.M. Corr (eds.). *Handbook of Childhood Death and Bereavement*, pp. 89-105. New York: Springer.

Faulkner, K.W. 1993. Children's understanding of death. In Armstrong-Daily, A. and S.Z. Golzer (eds.). *Hospice Care for Children*, pp. 9-21. New York: Oxford University Press.

———. 1997. Talking about death with a dying child. *American Journal of Nursing* 97(6): 64-69.

Gibbons, M.B. 1993. Psychosocial aspects of serious illness. In Armstrong-Daily, A. and S.Z. Golzer (eds.). *Hospice Care for Children*, pp. 60-74. New York: Oxford University Press.

Hilden, J.M., J. Watterson, and J. Chrastek. 2000. Tell the children. *Journal of Clinical Oncology* 18(17): 3193-3195.

Hilden, J. et al. 2001. Attitudes and practices among pediatric oncologists regarding end of life care: results of the 1998 American society of clinical oncology survey. *Journal of Clinical Oncology* 19(1): 205-212.

Hinds, P.S., L. Oakes, and W. Furman. 2001. End of life decision making in pediatric oncology. In Ferrell, B.R. and N. Coyle (eds.). 2001. *Textbook of Palliative Nursing*. New York: Oxford University Press.

Lauer, M.E. et al. 1989. Long term follow up of parental adjustment following a child's death at home or hospital. *Cancer* 63:988-994.

Martinson, I.M. 1995. Improving care of dying children. *Western Journal of Medicine* 163(3):258-262.

McGrath, P.A. (ed.). 1990. *Pain in Children: Nature, Assessment, and Treatment.* New York: The Guilford Press.

Miser, J.S. and A.W. Miser. 1993. Pain and symptom control in hospice care for children. In Armstrong-Daily, A. and S.Z. Golzer (eds.). *Hospice Care for Children,* pp. 22-59. New York: Oxford University Press.

National Hospice and Palliative Care Organization (NHPCO). 2000. *Compendium of Pediatric Palliative Care.* Alexandria, VA:NHPCO.

Other Resources: Websites

American Academy of Pediatrics (AAP). Palliative Care for Children. Found at www.aap.org. Includes a statement on principles of palliative care for children.

Childrens Hospice International (CHI). www.chionline.org

Cultural Sensitivity: Looking Through Different Eyes 9

I may be forced to adopt a new way of life, but my heart and spirit spring from the red earth.
— Painted Wolf (Doka and Davidson, 1998)

Making Room for Cultural Diversity

Mrs. Vang, a middle-aged Cambodian immigrant with advanced pancreatic cancer, is admitted to an oncology unit in extreme pain. Her family has not yet arrived at the hospital. When she is more comfortable, the doctor tries to talk with her about a DNR/DNI status but Mrs. Vang shakes her head. The oncology nurse sits down with her and says, "Please forgive me if I say anything that might be offensive to you. I'm trying to understand your needs so we can give you the best care possible." Mrs. Vang nods and says, "I need my family first. Then we can make decisions."

In America, we live in a kaleidoscope of cultural, social, ethnic, and religious beliefs that influence how each person looks at dying. As nurses caring for dying patients, it's important to acknowledge that our view of death and dying might be very different from that of our patients and their families.

For example, our American medical practices place a high value on the concept of individual patient autonomy and the patient's right to know about his or her diagnosis. We stress the importance of communicating directly with patients and of telling them the diagnosis. In contrast, physicians in Japan and Italy do not routinely tell their patients if they have a cancer diagnosis. This is the accepted and expected practice (Koenig and Gates-Williams 1995).

With our emphasis on the importance of individual rights, we expect patients to make their own decisions on treatment options. Yet, in many cultural groups, decision making is a group or family process (MDH 1996). Consider the mounting frustration of a hospice nurse caring for an immigrant patient from Southeast Asia. The patient was in extreme pain. In a discussion with her supervisor about the patient's mounting pain, the nurse said, "I keep telling the wife to give him morphine on a regular basis. I don't know why she won't listen to me." With further exploration, the nurse discovered that the wife was not the primary decision maker in this situation. The elders of the family directed the patient's care. Once the nurse spoke with the elders about the patient's pain and they agreed with her suggestions, the wife was able to start giving the morphine on a regular basis.

Our health care system is based on a scientific biomedical model of disease. Many other cultures have a more spiritual or nature-based view. For example, some Native Americans see illness as an imbalance between the heart, mind, body, and soul. Rather than looking for pharmaceutical or surgical remedies, they might look instead to a spiritual healer (Showalter 1998).

Others might view our system with mistrust because of past or current experience. For example, a number of studies of African-American communities have revealed mistrust for the system for a variety of reasons including a perception that medical treatment is less rigorous, clinics have a patronizing attitude toward them, and communication is not clear. Because of this, African Americans are sometimes more reluctant to forego aggressive treatment at the end of life (Barrett 1998).

Many of the culturally diverse patients and families we care for at the end of life have the added stressors of limited financial resources and health coverage. Culturally sensitive care includes taking these issues into consideration. Make use of the health team resources such as the social worker or patient advocate to provide the best care possible.

Understand Your Own Beliefs

In the previous situation with the nurse who encountered difficulties relieving her patient's pain, the nurse also discovered that she carried her own values and beliefs into the home. As she later told her supervisor, "It made me angry that the wife couldn't make decisions for herself."

When looking at culturally sensitive care for dying patients, look at your own attitudes, beliefs, and practices. (See sidebar, Questions to Ask Yourself About Your Own Attitudes and Beliefs.)

The ability to know yourself will give you insight on how you might respond to someone whose answers are different from your own. For example, if you feel strongly about the importance of disclosure in the case of a terminal illness, you know you need to step back and listen carefully to the family that requests that a patient not be told of the diagnosis.

In another example, you may believe that a "good death" means dying peacefully at home surrounded by family. Yet, this is not a universal concept. Some Chinese immigrants choose to avoid death at home because they believe that the ghost of the person who died will inhabit the home (Koenig and Gates-Williams 1995).

Listen to the Patients

With the variety and complexity of cultural differences within our society, it's not possible to *know* everything about each patient's beliefs and needs. The best approach you can take is one of honesty and active listening. It is okay to say, "I do not know much about your culture and beliefs, but I want to learn from you so I can give you the best care possible" (Showalter 1998).

Several approaches can help you to be an effective listener (MDH 1996):

▌ **Ask open-ended questions rather than questions that can be answered "yes" or "no."** This allows for discussion. For example, instead of asking, "Did you sleep well last night?" ask, "Tell me how you slept last night."
▌ **Be patient.** Sometimes a seemingly roundabout response to a question can yield valuable information.
▌ **Acknowledge the patient's perception of the illness.** If a patient says, "I believe a bad spirit has gotten into my stomach," instead of saying, "No, it's a bacterial infection," try, "Tell me more about it."

Listening to patients also means paying close attention to nonverbal communication. This includes facial expressions, eye contact, and touch. Evidence exists that facial expressions of emotions are universal (Andrews and Boyle 1995). If a patient appears to be in distress, take that as a cue that he/she *is* in distress. You can validate your observation by simply saying, "You look sad or uncomfortable or in pain."

Eye contact can be a misinterpreted nonverbal signal. In the majority of American society, it is the accepted practice to make direct eye contact when you look at people. However, in some Asian and Native American cultures, it is considered disrespectful to look directly at a person you consider a superior. This could easily be misinterpreted in our culture as someone who is either not listening or not interested. If you are talking with a patient or family and they are not looking directly at you, clarify, "Do you understand what I am saying?"

Because touch has a wide variety of meanings, it is always reasonable to ask, for example, "Is it all right if I hold your hand, or hug you, or stroke your forehead?" Not all people welcome human touch. For example, some Asian cultures believe that strength resides in a person's head; to touch the head is a sign of great disrespect (Andrews and Boyle 1995, p. 69).

Avoid Stereotyping and Making Assumptions

No magical formula exists for understanding various cultures. Culture is not homogenous, and you will find a great deal of diversity among individuals even in the smallest cultural group. Beware of stereotyping or making assumptions based on general knowledge of a patient's culture rather than a specific knowledge of the patient. For example, because you know that certain Asian cultures believe that patients should not be told of a terminal diagnosis, this does not mean you should assume that all Asian patients feel this way. The important thing to do is ask. "How much would you like to know about your illness?" (See sidebar, Ways to Avoid Cultural Stereotyping.)

Use Trained Medical Interpreters

Caring for patients when you encounter a language barrier is one of the most challenging aspects of working with a culturally diverse population. It's important to engage trained medical interpreters whenever possible. Do not use family members or people who are not trained in medical interpretation unless it is absolutely necessary. Oftentimes in an immigrant family children learn English before parents or grandparents and are asked to interpret. Not only are they not trained in medical language,

---

Ways To Avoid Cultural Stereotyping

▪ Prepare the patient for your questions by saying, "I am not very familiar with your customs. Please tell me if I ask questions that are offensive to you."

▪ Ask open-ended questions. Instead of asking, "Do you want your family here while I talk with you?" try, "Who else would you like to have here while I talk with you?"

▪ Ask patients and families to help you identify resources that will enhance your understanding of their care needs: "Who in your community could help me better understand how to best care for you?"

but asking them to interpret places a heavy and sometimes embarrassing burden of responsibility on them. As one teenage boy said, "How could I ask my grandmother about the private parts of her body?"

When using trained interpreters, consider the following suggestions (Andrews and Boyle 1995, p. 71):

■ Know the language your patient speaks before you engage an interpreter. Do not assume that people from the same country speak the same language.
■ Avoid an interpreter from rival tribes, regions, or nations.
■ Engage an interpreter of the same gender as the patient.
■ Speak to the patient, not the interpreter.

In reality, it is not always possible to use a trained medical interpreter. If you must communicate with a patient or family without the aid of an interpreter, do not raise your voice. Speak in a low, moderate voice using a polite and formal tone. You can also try:

■ Using simple words. Instead of discomfort, use pain.
■ Asking direct questions such as "Are you in pain?"
■ Giving instructions in simple language and demonstrating them. "Put the medicine into the dropper like this. Then place it in his cheek like this."
■ Discussing one topic at a time. Do not ask, "Are you having trouble breathing or sleeping at night?"

Whenever possible, identify resources to help you with the language barrier. Look for materials written in the patient's language. Find someone in the community who can help you with simple phrases.

Use Community Resources

Many communities of diversity have their own "cultural informants." These are people from within the community who are able to interact with the larger American society. Cultural informants can be invaluable both to help you better understand the needs of your patient and to help you link the patient with community programs.

Advocating for Patients and Families

If you work in a health care institution, look at the policies of your workplace regarding cultural sensitivity. Do you have trained interpreters available? Do you have written resources for your patients in their own language? Are your policies flexible enough to accommodate patients and families of diverse backgrounds? To work toward a culturally supportive place for patients and families to be at the end of life consider:

- Creating space to accommodate extended families.
- Instituting nonrestrictive visiting hours. An Asian-American daughter said of her mother's death, "In my family, we do not believe people should die alone. When my mother was in the hospital, they made us go home for the night. She died alone. They said that when they found her, she had tears in her eyes. I will live with that always."
- Allowing important rituals such as a traditional healing ceremony.
- Routinely asking how the family prefers the body to be treated. For example, an Islamic family might request that the body be turned to the east at the time of death (Koenig and Gates-Williams 1995). Or another family might request the opportunity to bathe and prepare the body after death.

Summary

Working with patients and families of different cultural, ethnic, religious, and socio-economic backgrounds during the last steps of a journey in life is an art. It's the art of being aware of diverse needs, the art of listening, and the art of balancing your own culture and the culture of your institution with the culture of the patient and family.

References

Andrews, M.A. and J.S. Boyle. 1995. *Transcultural Concepts of Nursing Care.* Philadelphia, PA: J.B. Lippincott, pp. 67-71.

Barrett, R.K. 1998. Sociocultural considerations for working with blacks. In Doka, K.J. and J.D. Davidson. *Living with Grief.* Washington, DC: Hospice Foundation of America, pp. 83-96.

DeSpelder, L.A. 1998. Developing cultural competency. In Doka, K.J. and J.D. Davidson. *Living with Grief.* Washington, DC: Hospice Foundation of America, pp. 97-106.

Doka, K.J. and J.D. Davidson. 1998. *Living with Grief.* Washington, DC: Hospice Foundation of America,

Koenig, B. and J. Gates-Williams. 1995. Understanding cultural difference in caring for dying patients. *Western Journal of Medicine* 163(3): 244-248.

Minnesota Department of Health (MDH). 1996. *Six Steps Toward Cultural Competence.* Refugee Health Program. Minneapolis, MN: MDH.

Showalter, S.E. 1998. Looking through different eyes: Beyond cultural diversity. In Doka, K.J. and J.D. Davidson. *Living with Grief.* Washington, DC: Hospice Foundation of America, pp. 71-82.

Other Resources

Books

Ferrell, B.R. and N. Coyle (eds.). 2001. *Textbook of Palliative Nursing.* New York: Oxford University Press.

Geissler, E.M. 1998. *A Pocket Guide to Cultural Assessment.* St. Louis: Mosby.

Website

Office of Minority Health Resource Center. Washington, DC: Department of Health and Human Services. www.omhrc.gov. Includes links to state organizations and resources.

Hospice: The Gold Standard for End of Life Care 10

Hospice adds life to days when days can no longer be added to life.

— The Family Handbook of Hospice Care

A Philosophy of Care

George is a 78-year-old man who lives in a senior citizen's high-rise with his 76-year-old wife. Five days ago he suffered a severe stroke. He is currently hospitalized on a neurology floor and is minimally responsive. His wife and family have chosen not to pursue any further aggressive treatment for him including the insertion of a feeding tube. The family asks the nurse, "What do we do now?" She says, "What do you know about hospice care?" The wife looks concerned and says, "But George didn't want to be put someplace. He always wanted to be at home." The nurse then explains that hospice can help the family take George home and care for him there. The nurse discusses the family prefer-ence to care for the patient at home with the physician and obtains an order for hospice care. The nurse then arranges a conference with the family, the social worker, and a hos-pice coordinator to discuss discharge plans.

In order to explain hospice to your patients and families, you need to understand the basic philosophy of hospice care. The focus of hospice is on ensuring that a pa-tient's remaining days are comfortable. It is considered the gold standard of care for people at the end of life's journey. (See sidebar, Hospice Care.)

Most patients enrolled in hospice are able to spend their final days in the comfort of their own home. For those who cannot be at home, hospice care can be provided in a hospital, nursing home, or other type of residential setting.

The hospice philosophy of care embraces a holistic approach to the patient and family. The focus of care is on comfort and dignity for the patient and family during the last months, weeks, and days of the patient's life.

> **Hospice Care**
>
> ▪ Emphasizes living as fully as possible
> ▪ Provides relief from the physical, emotional, and spiritual distress that often accompany a life-limiting illness
> ▪ Provides support for the family while they are caring for their loved one
> ▪ Provides grief support for the family following the death

Who Qualifies for Hospice Care?

Hospice care is provided for patients who have a terminal diagnosis and are no longer pursuing active aggressive treatment to cure the disease. Most hospice programs use admission criteria established through the Hospice Medicare Benefit. In order to receive services patients need to:

▪ Have a diagnosis with a prognosis of six months or less as certified by a physician. This means that given the patient's disease and current status, the doctor expects that he/she will die within six months.
▪ Sign a hospice consent form agreeing to care that focuses on comfort rather than on either cure or treatments to prolong life.

Referral to hospice does not require a physician's order. However, a physician must be involved once a plan of care for the patient has been established.

Six-Month Prognosis

The six-month prognosis can sometimes be a barrier for referral to hospice. Physicians may be reluctant to predict that a patient will die in this period of time. If you feel a patient could benefit from hospice care, and the physician is unsure of the prognosis, remember, this time frame is only an estimate. While most patients enrolled in hospice live less than two months (NHPCO 2000), some continue to receive services much longer than six months. The hospice program will reevaluate the patient on a regular basis. Research has shown that physicians are more likely to overestimate a lifespan than underestimate it (Christakis and Lamont 2000). Consider approaching a reluctant physician with these two questions:

▪ Would you be surprised if this patient was still alive in six months?
▪ Is this patient sick enough to die?

Hospice Philosophy of Care

The second criterion for hospice admission, the patient agreeing to a hospice philosophy of care, can also be problematic. Hospices interpret the meaning of this differently. For example, some hospice programs will not admit patients who are receiving chemotherapy because they view this treatment as curative rather than palliative. If your patient is receiving specialized treatments, discuss these with the hospice admissions coordinator. If one program will not accept a patient, try another.

How Do I Approach Patients and Families About Hospice Care?

Patients who accept hospice care have crossed a very difficult bridge from looking to medical care for cure or for life extension to looking at life completion. Talking about hospice is not an easy conversation. The best approach is an honest one. "It looks like the course of your care is changing. I'd like to talk with you about hospice." Some patients and families will be willing and interested to learn more. Others will need time. And others will not consider hospice as an option. Listen carefully to their questions and provide as much information as they want. This is a good time to also engage other members of the team including the physician, social worker, and chaplain.

Common concerns when talking about hospice include:

- "Are you sure its time to talk about hospice? Can't we try some other treatments?" Review with the patient and family their understanding of the illness and the treatment options. Use simple and straightforward language to clarify their questions. Many treatment options are still available to patients receiving hospice care.
- "If we talk about hospice, the patient might give up hope." Clarify what is meant by "hope." For the seriously ill, hope can take on a dimension very different than one of cure. It can mean having the time to accomplish some goals such as saying good-bye or putting affairs in order. For some, hope means being at home. For others, hope is defined by feeling comforted and cared for.
- "Does this mean the doctor will quit treating?" Many patients feel they will be abandoned by their physicians if they agree to hospice care. Avoid saying, "There's nothing more we can do for you." Instead, reassure the patient that their physician will continue to direct care. Also assure them that many treatments still exist and will be used, but the focus will be on comfort and palliation, not cure.

The Hospice Medicare Benefit

Hospice care is covered under a special Medicare Benefit. It is also provided under Medicaid and private insurance companies. The Medicare Hospice Benefit covers:

- Medical and symptom management focused on enhancing comfort. Care is provided by a team of professionals including the patient's primary physician, nurses, and the hospice medical director.
- Emotional and spiritual care. Hospice care includes visits by social workers, chaplains, and volunteers.
- Coverage for medications, supplies, and medical equipment related to the terminal diagnosis
- Assistance with bathing, personal care, and homemaking
- Volunteer services for respite, companionship, errands
- Hospitalization for acute episodes. Extended hours of care in the home for acute episodes
- Respite care for times when the family is exhausted or unable to provide care
- Grief support for the family

In George's case (see beginning of the chapter) the hospice staff will help arrange for his discharge to home. This will include ordering a hospital bed and any other equipment the family might need to care for him in his apartment. He will receive regular visits from the hospice nurse to manage his physical care. A home health aide will be offered to help with George's bath and personal care. The hospice social worker will help his wife and family deal with some of the complexities of caring for a person at home. In addition the hospice chaplain will be available to discuss spiritual issues. Hospice volunteers will also be available to provide companionship, respite care, or run errands.

Hospice will provide the family with 24-hour call service. George will also be eligible for extended hours of care during a medical crisis. The goal of his care will be to provide the support to George and his family to keep him comfortable and in his apartment as long as possible. When George dies, the hospice program will follow up with his family, providing support and counseling up to one year after the death.

While hospice care under the Hospice Medicare Benefit is a comprehensive benefit, it does have limitations. It's important to be aware of those areas not covered under the benefit. (See sidebar, Hospice Medicare Benefit Limitations.)

Advocating for Your Patients

Most patients, when facing a life-limiting or terminal illness, prefer to be cared for in their own home. As an advocate, ask the patient and family, "Where would you like to be?" Hospice is a comprehensive program covered by insurance and Medicare that strives to keep patients in their own home as long as possible. Make sure you are aware of the hospice programs in your area. Have brochures and information available to your patients and families. Offer hospice care as an option. As a hospice director said, "One of the most common comments we receive on our family surveys is that we wish hospice had been offered sooner."

> **Hospice Medicare Benefit Limitations**
>
> ▌ Does not provide 24-hour caregiving services. Extended hours of care (continuous care) are available during a crisis. If a patient routinely needs 24-hour care that the family is unable to provide, the hospice social worker will assist the family in setting up services. These are generally private pay arrangements.
> ▌ Does not cover treatments and medications unrelated to the terminal illness. For example, if a patient is an insulin-dependent diabetic but the terminal diagnosis is lung cancer, hospice will not cover the cost of the insulin and related supplies.
> ▌ Does not cover curative or experimental treatments aimed at cure.

Summary

Hospice care is a philosophy of care that encompasses the complex physical, personal, family, and spiritual needs of a dying person. Care is provided by a team of health professionals including the patient's primary physician, a hospice nurse, social worker, chaplain, home health aides, volunteers, and others as needed. Under the Hospice Medicare Benefit, patients qualify for hospice if they have a terminal illness with a prognosis of six months or less and they choose a philosophy of care that emphasizes comfort over cure.

References

Christakis, N.A. and E.B. Lamont. 2000. Extent and determinants of error in doctors' prognosis in terminally ill patients: Prospective cohort study. *British Medical Journal* 320(7233):469-472.

National Hospice and Palliative Care Organization (NHPCO). Washington, DC. www.nhpco.org

Other Resources

The Family Handbook of Hospice Care. 1999. Minneapolis, MN: Fairview Press.

Hospice Care: A Physician's Guide. 2001. Washington, DC: National Hospice and Palliative Care Organization.

Lattanzi-Licht, M., J. Mahoney, and G. Miller. 1998. *The Hospice Choice.* New York: Fireside Books.

A Final Note: Taking Care 11

– To care for the dying, we must embrace our humanity.

– Walter Hunter, MD (Hamilton 2000)

Burning Brightly, Burning Dimly

Caring for patients who are at the end of life is one of the most difficult, yet reward-ing, experiences a nurse can have. It takes skill, wisdom, and courage to be present for the patient and for the patient's family at this crucial part of a person's life. You may experience the same doubts and fears that your patient does. You may find yourself agonizing over the questions about the meaning of life and hope. Some-times working with a dying patient will remind you of your own personal losses. To be present for your patients, you must also take care of yourself.

The late Frank Lamendola, RN, PhD, a nurse leader in end of life care, identified how our energy and compassion can ebb and flow. He called it burning brightly, burning dimly (Lamendola 1996). You will have those times when you feel you have given the best of yourself and your skills for the patient and the family. Those are the times of burning brightly. "You enter into the experience willingly and openly, not as a bystander, but as a participant in the lives of your patients and their families" (Lamendola 1996, p.16R).

And you will have the times of burning dimly. Those are the days when you're overly fatigued and find it's hard to give compassionately of yourself. A hospice nurse said it well the day she reported to her supervisor, "I can't take one more sad story. I have no more tears left."

During those times when you burn dimly, step back and give yourself a breather. If you are feeling "worn out," consider ways that are renewing for you. Some nurses use meditation, relaxation, exercise, or journaling. If you are struggling with the spiritual issues around meaning and existence, perhaps this is a good time to seek guidance from your own faith community, a chaplain, or a trusted colleague. Also consider what you can do within your institution or agency. Some hospital units, nursing homes, or home health agencies have regular memorial services or staff retreats to remember patients and recognize the work you and other staff have done.

Living in the Present Moment

Just as every human being is unique, every dying experience is unique. You have the opportunity to experience remarkable spiritual and emotional fulfillment when your patient dies well. But, despite your best care and efforts, not all your patients will die well. When you are a part of a difficult dying experience or a difficult death, avoid looking at it as a failure and second-guessing the care you have provided. A hospice nurse said of her first year of caring for dying patients, "I drove myself crazy when things didn't go well. I'd ask myself, 'What if I had upped the dose of morphine? Maybe I should have called the chaplain sooner. Why wasn't I there when the patient died?' I nearly burned out until a wiser, more experienced nurse took me aside and said, 'Look at the good things you did in that case. Give yourself credit and allow yourself to move on.'"

If you have an experience that does not go well or that drains you, take some time to reflect on it. What can you learn? How will this knowledge pave the way for the next patient? Consider this wisdom a gift. Then plant yourself firmly in the present for the patients you are caring for now and say, "I can do this, I am strong."

The Joy and the Laughter

Dr. Walter Hunter, a hospice medical director says about working with the dying, "Laughter and joy can be a more effective medicine than anything we hope to produce in the laboratory" (Hamilton 2001). Remember, those who are dying are also living, and laughter is a part of living.

Consider the story a hospice coordinator tells of a 67-year-old woman who was at home and nearing death.

"I received a call from her very distraught son. He asked, 'When is Mom going to die?' I'd never met the patient so I asked him some questions about her. He told me he was calling because his mother had gathered them to the bedside in the morning to tell them good-bye. 'But, she hasn't died yet and I don't know if something is wrong.' I told him I'd have a nurse come out to visit and that I'd call him right away in the morning to see how things were going. The next day I called. He started to laugh when I asked how things were. 'Well,' he said. 'Mom gathered us all to the bedside again last night. She apologized for saying good-bye too soon. We didn't quite know what to say until she started to laugh and said, 'Of course, I've never done this before, so how would I know?' The son said it was a wonderful moment for the family. 'In all the worry about Mom dying, we'd forgotten how to laugh.' The patient died very peacefully two days later."

A Final Note

Caring for people at the end of life is the essence of nursing. We have the opportunity to witness and nurture the richness and grace of the human spirit in those final days and hours. Use this book to find out what you "don't know." Then use the resources listed to build something solid to stand upon so you can be present for your patients and families. Dr. Elisabeth Kubler-Ross said, "Taking care of terminal patients is a privilege and a gift which teaches us not only about dying, but about living" (Kubler-Ross 1999, p. 34).

References

Hamilton, C. 2001. Caring for the seriously ill: 12 ethical imperatives for working with the dying. *Supportive Voice Newsletter of Supportive Care of the Dying* 7(2):4-5.

Kubler-Ross, E. 1999. In *The Family Handbook of Hospice Care*. Minneapolis, MN: Fairview Press.

Lamendola, F. 1996. Keeping your compassion alive. *American Journal of Nursing* 96(11): 16R-16T.

Index

A

Active dying (care near death), 47–54
  breathing changes, 49
  children and, 66
  clinical indicators, 48–51
  communicating, 52–53
  consciousness levels, 50
  family needs, 51–53
  food and fluid changes, 48–49
  interventions, 49, 50, 51
  interventions to avoid, 52
  life-sustaining treatments, 53
  pain, 51
  patient needs, 51–53
  phrases helpful in , 52
  resources, 54
  skin changes, 50
Acute care settings, 15, 25
Adolescent care, 64
Adjuvant medication in pain management, 23
Advance care planning, 9–17
  advance directives, 10, 12–13
  barriers to, 12–13
  communication in, 10, 12, 14–15
  elements of, 10–12
  family needs, 12, 14, 15
  patient needs, 11–12, 13, 15–16
  phrases helpful in, 14
  questions about, 15–16
  resources, 12, 17
Advance directives, 10, 12–13
  questions about, 15–16
  wills and, 15
Advocate role of nurses, *x*, 3
  active dying, 51–52
  advance care planning, 13
  after-death care, 57
  cultural diversity, 75–76
  hospice care, 82

  pain and assessment management, 24–25
  pediatric care, 66–67
  physical symptom management, 35–36
  suffering, 42–43
After death (care of families), 55–61
  children and loss, 58–59
  communicating, 56, 58, 59
  grief, 55–57
  loss and acceptance, 57–59
  phrases to avoid, 59
  resources, 60–61
  self-care for nurses, 60
Alcohol dependency, 33
Alternative therapies. *See* Complementary and
    integrative therapies
Anticonvulsants, 23
Antidepressants, 23, 35
Anti-inflammatory drugs, 23
Anxiety, 34
  in children, 66
Appetite loss, 33
Attorneys and advance care planning, 12, 15–16

B

Breathing problems, 30–31, 49
  with children, 66

C

Care settings, 5
  home, 4, 43, 68
  hospice, 24, 36, 43, 79–83
  hospital, 15, 25
  pain management and, 24–25
  suffering and, 43
Chaplains, 5, 6, 13, 15, 57
Chemical dependency, 33
Children
  death of, 64–65
  loss and, 58–59
  See also Pediatric end of life care

Clergy, 5, 13, 15
Clinician role of nurses, *x*, 3
    active dying, 47–51
    advance care planning, 10–12
    after-death care, 55–57
    pain and assessment management, 20–24
    pediatric care, 65–66
    physical symptom management, 30–35
    suffering, 40–42
Communications
    in active dying, 52–53
    in advance care planning, 10, 12, 14–15
    cultural sensitivity issues, 74–75
    hospice care, 81
    in pain assessment and management, 20, 21–22, 24
    in pediatric care, 65, 66–67
    in physical symptom management, 36
Complementary and integrative therapies, 21, 23–24, 52
Consciousness changes near death, 50
    in children, 66
Constipation, 32
Corticosteroids, 23
Counselors, 5
Cultural considerations, 57, 71–77
    communicating, 74–75
    cultural stereotypes, 74
    family and patient needs, 75–76
    medical interpreters, 74–75
    nurses beliefs, 72–73
    pain management, 24–25

D
Depression, 23, 34–35
Diarrhea, 32
Dietician, 6
DNR/DNI orders, 12–13
Durable health care power of attorney, 12
Dyspnea, 31–32

F
Family needs and preferences, 3–4
    active dying, 51–53
    advance care planning, 12, 14, 15
    after death, 55–59
    pain assessment and management, 21–22, 24–26
    pediatric care, 66–69
    suffering, 41–42, 43–45

    See also After death (care of families)
Fatigue, 34, 48
Food and fluid intake, 48–49

G
Grief and loss, 3, 55–60
    See also After death (care of families)
Guide role of nurses, *x*, 3
    active dying, 52–53
    advance care planning, 13–15
    after-death care, 57–59
    pain and assessment management, 25–27
    pediatric care, 68–69
    physical symptom management, 36
    suffering, 44–45

H
Health care agents, 12, 16
Health care directives, 10, 12
    See also Advance directives
Health care proxies, 12
Holistic aspects of care, 4, 6, 42–43
Home care settings, 4, 43
    for children, 68
Hospice care, 24, 36, 43, 79–83
    communicating, 81
    Medicare Benefit for, 81–82, 83
    patient preferences, 82
    philosophy of care, 79, 80–81
    qualifying for, 80–81
    resources, 83
Hospital care settings, 15, 25

I
Infant and toddler care, 63–64
Integrative therapies. *See* Complementary and integrative therapies
Intubation and advance directives, 12–13

L
Language barriers and medical interpreters, 74–75
Language to avoid
    after death, 59
pain management, 20
Language to use
    active dying, 52
    advance care planning, 14
Lawyers and advance care planning, 12, 15–16
Life-sustaining treatments, 53

Living wills, 10, 12
    See also Advance directives
Loss and grief, 3, 55–60

M

Medical interpreters and language barriers, 74–75
Medicare Benefit for hospice care, 81–82, 83
Medications, 22–23, 35, 43, 50
    pediatric, 65, 66
    narcotic addiction misconceptions, 25– 26

N

Narcotic addiction misconceptions, 25– 26
Nausea and vomiting, 33
Near-death care. *See* Active dying
NSAIDS (nonsteroidal anti-inflammatory drugs), 23
Nursing assessments, 4–5
    active dying, 47–51
    pain, 20–22
    pediatric care, 65–66
    physical symptom management, 31–35
    suffering, 39–43
Nursing care (end of life), 1–6
    active dying, 47–54
    after death, 55–61
    advance care planning, 9–17
    cultural considerations, 71–77
    hospice care, 79–83
    pain assessment and management, 19–28
    pediatric care, 63–70
    physical symptom management, 29–37
    principles for, 2, 3
    self care, 85–87
    start of, 4–5
    suffering, 39–45
    See also Nursing assessments; Nursing interventions
Nursing interventions
    active dying, 49, 50, 51, 52
    complementary therapies, 21, 23– 24, 52
    pain, 22–23, 25
    pediatric care, 65, 66
    physical symptom management, 31, 32, 33, 34, 35
    suffering, 43
Nursing roles and responsibilities, *ix–x*, 2– 3
    See also Advocate role of nurses; Clinician role of nurses; Guide role of nurses

P

Pain assessment and management, 2–4, 19–28
    active dying, 50, 51
    adjuvant medication, 23
    assessment basics, 20–22
    for children, 65
    communicating in, 20, 21–22, 24
    complementary and integrative therapies, 23–24
    family needs, 21–22, 24–26
    interventions, 22–23, 25
    management principles, 22
    medications, 22– 23, 25
    misconceptions, 25–26
    patient needs, 21–22, 24–26
    pediatric care, 65
    phrases to avoid, 20
    principles, 22
    resources, 26–27, 28
    suffering compared, 40
Palliative care, 2, 4, 5
Patient needs and preferences, 3–4
    active dying, 51–53
    advance care planning, 11–13, 15–16
    cultural sensitivity, 75–76
    DNR/DNI orders, 12–13
    hospice care, 82
    pain assessment and management, 21–22, 24–26
    pediatric care, 66–69
    physical symptom management, 35–36
    suffering, 41–42, 43–45
Pediatric end of life care, 64–70
    active dying, 66
    characteristics, 64
    communicating, 65, 66–67
    family and patient needs, 66–69
    medications, 65, 66
    pain, 65
    physicians, 67–68
    resources, 69–70
    symptoms, 65–66
Personal suffering, 41–42
Physical symptom management, 2, 29–37
    assessment, 30–35
    children, 65–66
    common symptoms, 30, 31–35
    communicating in, 36
    interventions, 31, 32, 33, 34, 35
    patient and family needs, 35–36

Physical symptom management *(continued)*
  pediatric, 65–66
  resources, 37
  suffering, 40–41
Physicians, 5–6
  advance care planning, 13, 14
  pediatric care, 67–68
Power of attorney, 12
Preparations for dying, 3, 4
  See also Active dying
Proxies for health care decisions, 12

R
Religion. *See* Spiritual care
Resuscitation and advance directives, 12–13
Risk for dying (symptoms), 4–5

S
School-age child's care, 64
Self care for nurses and caregivers, 60, 85–87
Self knowledge (nurse)
  cultural sensitivity and, 72–73
  suffering and, 43–44
Skilled clinician role. *See* Clinician role of
  nurses
Skin disorders, 33–34, 50
Social workers, 6, 13, 41, 57

Spiritual care
  cultural issues, 72
  providers, 5, 6, 13, 15, 57
  spiritual suffering, 42
Suffering, 3, 39–45
  communicating in care of, 41–42, 43–45
  family and patient needs, 41–42, 43–45
  holistic view, 42–43
  nurse self-assessment, 43–44
  pain compared, 40
  personal, 41–42
  physical, 40–41
  spiritual, 42
Symptom management. *See* Physical symptom
  management
Symptoms of risk for dying, 4–5

T
Team approach to care, 5–6, 15
Toddler and infant care, 63–64

V
Vomiting and nausea, 33

W
Weight loss, 33
Wills and advance directives, 15